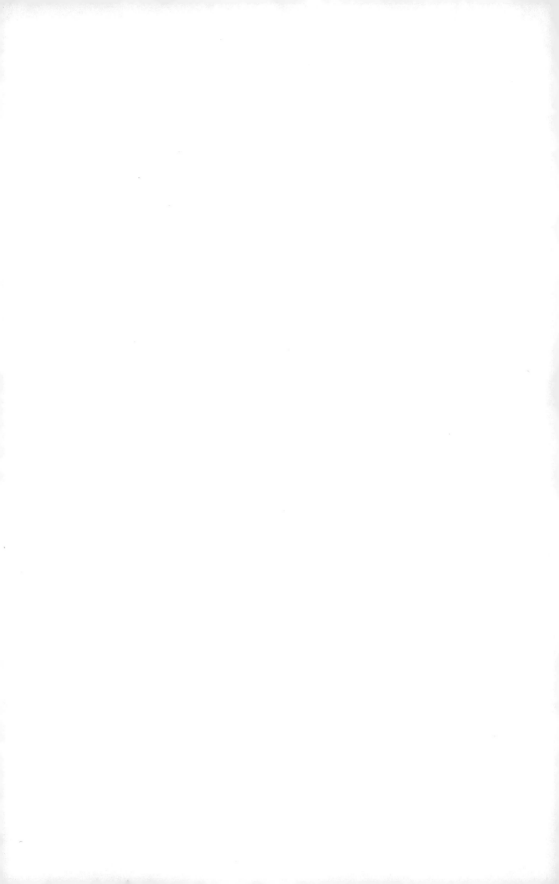

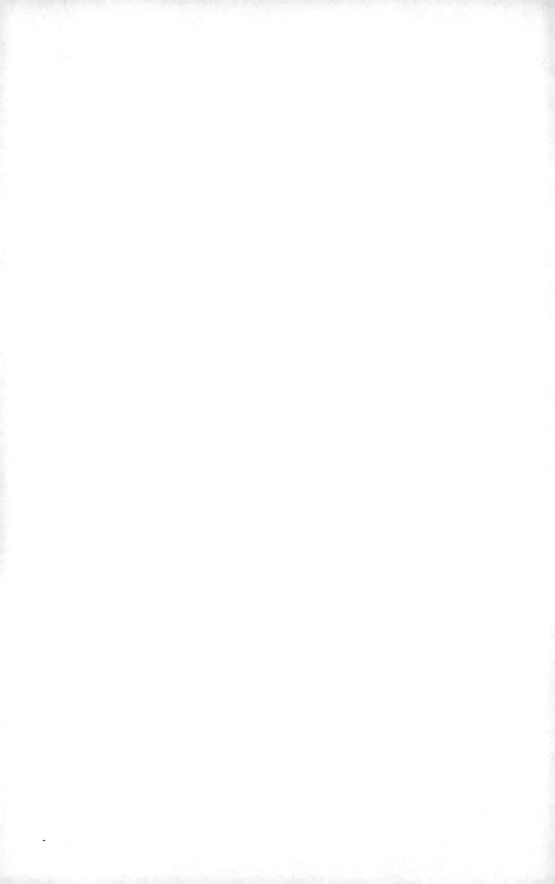

MEDICINE WORTH PAYING FOR

Medicine Worth Paying For

Assessing Medical Innovations

Edited by

Howard S. Frazier and
Frederick Mosteller

Harvard University Press
Cambridge, Massachusetts
London, England
1995

Library of Congress Cataloging-in-Publication Data

Medicine worth paying for : assessing medical innovations / edited by
Howard S. Frazier and Frederick Mosteller.
p.   cm.
Includes bibliographical references and index.
ISBN 0-674-56362-X
1. Medical innovations—Evaluation.   2. Medical innovations—Case
studies.   3. Medical innovations—Economic aspects.   I. Frazier,
Howard S., 1926–   .   II. Mosteller, Frederick, 1916–
RA418.5.M4M425   1995
610′ .068′5—dc20
94-48899

43.00

The editors dedicate this book to Lenore Frazier and Virginia Mosteller, both of whom have viewed our piles of paper and our preoccupations with forbearance and good humor

Contents

Preface

Describing how a book came to be written can easily become an exercise in creative recollection. In this instance, however, certain of the book's preconditions, accidents of time and place, or careful plans of colleagues loom so large as to guide recall.

Surely one seminal influence is that of Howard H. Hiatt, who, installed in 1972 as the Dean of the Harvard School of Public Health, brought to his new post the conviction that the health and health care of populations were so complex as to invite the best efforts not of physicians alone but of problem-oriented, multidisciplinary teams of investigators. This idea was first embodied in the Faculty Seminar, an array of working groups whose members came from universities, state and local governments, teaching hospitals, and consulting firms. In its formative period, the Seminar was led first by Fred Mosteller and then by John Bunker. They were able to organize, nurture, and focus the efforts of a rich collection of talent just becoming accustomed to unfamiliar subjects and styles of work.

Of equal importance to the success of the venture was the willingness of a number of foundations to support, over the past twenty years, a variety of activities that at best were unconventional and, as the intellectual life of the Seminar became more intense, may at times have seemed close to tumult.

From the standpoint of organizational structure, the Faculty Seminar spawned a series of working groups that have continued to meet, work, and write, some for as long as twenty years. From the standpoint of organizational culture, the Faculty Seminar established a tradition of research collaboration across disciplinary boundaries that continues to facilitate our work and encourages us to address problems clearly beyond our reach as individual investigators.

We have chosen the method of multiple case studies to illustrate both the benefits of medicine and the themes of the book. The method has the advantage of concreteness and therefore of relevance to real life. In addition, by documenting the effectiveness of successful innovations, a collection of case studies gives us some idea of the amount of good being done by successful medical innovations in general. We also learn from the similarities between cases, for example, the importance of promptly evaluating new technologies and of enlisting a wide range of individuals as subjects. Even the best therapies have shortcomings, and studying the outcomes of different innovations allows us to suggest methods to improve their performance and the performance of others like them.

Although the number of our cases is modest, we have been able to include examples from medicine, surgery, pharmaceuticals, dentistry, public health, and even organizational innovation. Each case has implications for public policy, especially for achievable changes in policy. We have emphasized the implications that will be useful no matter what form the health care system takes on in the near future. Where solutions to problems are not apparent, we hope that the cases will serve to open debate.

Before presenting the case studies, we provide in Part A a brief introduction to the field of technology assessment. In Chapter 1 we discuss what it means to ask, and answer, a very important question: "How is medicine doing?" In Chapter 2 we outline the main methods of assessing medical technologies and give some notion of the strengths and limitations of the methods, especially the method of randomized clinical trials.

The fourteen case studies are gathered together into eight sections (Parts B–I) focusing on different aspects of the health care system: physician performance; perverse financial incentives; patient empowerment; monitoring and delivering health care; the maintenance of visual and dental health; quality of life; unanticipated effects of medical treatment; and innovations in the administration of health care. To emphasize the common themes of the cases, we have supplied introductory notes for each of these parts. Following each case study we have added an editorial note summarizing the implications of the particular study for the health care system in general. In order to lighten the text a bit, we include vignettes illustrating related issues set off from the main text.

The final part brings together our conclusions and suggestions for change. In Chapter 17 we outline a number of programs being developed to improve the assessment of the health care system. These proposals are of particular interest because they are relatively independent of the type of health care system that will actually be adopted. In Chapter 18 we summarize the findings from the cases and from the development of new, innovation-specific programs. We then combine both the general and specific recommendations in Chapter 19.

We hope that anyone with an interest in the problems of supplying health care to the nation will find our case studies useful. Because we hope to reach readers without a medical education, we have encouraged our authors to go easy on the technical vocabulary of medicine and where possible to use everyday language. So although many physicians will find much that interests them in this book, they are not expected to learn new medicine here.

We have limited the number of references, giving preference to those that the non-physician reader will find most helpful. We do include some key references to the primary research literature as well. We want to be sure that physicians appreciate the need for technology assessment at every level and that they recognize how frequently good ideas with support from basic research in biology have turned out not to work in the clinical setting. We do want, however, to maintain some faith in the continuity of science and medicine, the scientific basis for ideas that contribute to good medical care.

We believe that the lessons embedded in the innovations we describe will interest a variety of readers, particularly those concerned with health policy, investigators studying health services, those in the health professions, laity who wish to improve the performance of the health care system for themselves as well as for all of us, and others who simply want health services that provide benefits greater than risks at an acceptable financial cost.

An enterprise of this sort depends heavily on bibliographic skills. We are grateful to Bruce Kupelnick, Carol Surridge, and Michele Orza for their assistance. In addition, Michele Orza gave liberally of her expertise on many aspects of oral contraceptives during the course of this study. Elisabeth Burdick offered advice and help throughout the preparation of this volume, in addition to her contributions as author.

In kneading our manuscript into the form of a book, we were greatly helped by the skills, experience, and enthusiasm of Kate Schmit at Harvard University Press.

On March 22, 1993, in a paper entitled "Some Evaluation Needs" at the Conference on Doing More Good Than Harm sponsored by the New York Academy of Sciences, Mosteller included some of the ideas presented in Chapter 17. Mosteller and Frazier, in a paper invited by the *Journal of the Italian Statistical Society* entitled "Improving the Contributions of Technology Assessment," presented in the fall of 1993 some of the findings from the case studies described in Chapter 18. The portions of Chapters 17 and 18 that were written for these conferences appear with the permission of the sponsoring organizations.

The editors and other contributors to this study take particular pleasure in thanking the Andrew W. Mellon Foundation and the Alfred P. Sloan Foundation for their support of the preparation of this book.

PART A

Background

1

The Nature of the Enquiry

HOWARD S. FRAZIER AND FREDERICK MOSTELLER

How Is Medicine Doing?

Being sick is hard and sometimes dangerous work. It elicits fears of death, pain, disability, and abandonment. To a great extent we allay these fears by putting our trust in modern medicine: we trust our caregivers to understand what is wrong with us, to know how and when to intervene, and to be available in our times of need. Is this faith in medical intervention justified? More specifically, how do we decide whether a particular drug or procedure is beneficial?

This important question—what works and what doesn't—has not received much dispassionate, empirically based analysis until very recently. The reasons for this apparent neglect are many. Comfort can be derived from having faith in the benefits of medicine, whether or not that faith is warranted. Furthermore, information on the outcomes of medical practices tends to be fragmentary, and medicine has few accepted methods for combining existing information from several sets of observations in order to make more powerful inferences. Finally, many people believe or assume that it is not important to know about the differential benefits of medical interventions because society can and will pay for any treatment that might be considered potentially advantageous.

That comfortable set of expectations has changed. The pace of development of new patterns of care has accelerated, exposing some caregivers as archaic and fallible. In addition, all of us have conflicting feelings about being under a doctor's care: on the one hand we want to be dependent, to be cared *for,* and on the other we insist on understanding the technical content of our care and participating in its selection. Frustrated by these contradictions between care and control, many have sought relief either in aimless doctor-bashing or in equally uncritical enthusiasm for the cornucopia of new and largely untried medical technologies.

How, in fact, is medicine doing at the end of the twentieth century? The question is an important one from a variety of perspectives, including the following three. First, caregivers are commanded by their codes of ethics to avoid doing harm. This implies an obligation to understand enough about cause and effect to avoid treatments that have negative consequences unless they offer a countervailing advantage to the patient. Second, we now recognize that the societal resources available for health care are limited. That being so, we ought to spend those resources on treatments that are likely to work. And third, the information needed to address the first two issues—how not to do harm, how not to waste resources—is costly to gather and interpret, and research money comes from the same pool of resources that is devoted to health care. The costs of learning how to guide the delivery of care, then, are competing with the direct costs of care itself. What pattern of resource allocation best serves our conflicting needs to determine what works and at the same time provide care to those who need it? Our own conviction is that, in general, it is cheaper and less risky to pay the cost of learning what works and what doesn't than to continue to deliver treatments whose risks and benefits seem reasonable but are unproven.

Many treatments widely accepted for use in health care have not received credible study of their risks and benefits when used under optimal conditions or under average conditions. Even when one knows the results of such studies for a series of alternative treatments, it may be difficult to choose the one best fitted to both individual and societal preferences. Sometimes those preferences will be opposed, because the best choice for society as a whole is usually to do some good for the most people whereas the best choice for an individual is usually to do the most good for just that one person. Gaining the knowledge on which we must base our selection of the best alternative is the goal of the field of study called *technology assessment.*

The Variety of Outcomes

One task of technology assessment is to evaluate the efficacy of treatments: What are the risks and benefits of interventions? This leaves open the question of exactly what risks and which benefits. What do we want an intervention to be able to do? At one time, the answer to this question would have been short and simple: it would prevent death. Both the capabilities of health care and our expectations of it have expanded beyond this criterion. Now we are likely to ask not only about mortality but about a variety of outcomes of treatment: morbidity (roughly, the persistence of limited function due to disease), stabilization or restoration of function, pain, the financial impact of treatment and its time horizon, patient satisfaction, overall quality of life, and the many possible adverse events or unwanted side effects related to the treatment itself.

Evaluation is impeded by two features of these outcomes. First, we lack a simple, common yardstick that puts outcomes for a group of people on a single scale. For example, imagine that total hip replacement for the treatment of painful, degenerative arthritis of the hip on average is successful in improving the patient's condition but, on average, reduces life expectancy because of complications related to the surgery. At present, analysts have no easy, generally accepted way to collapse the information about relief of symptoms and risk of dying into a single figure of merit for the treatment that lets them compare it with other treatments for the same problem. Without a common measure, it is difficult to say how individuals or society value a treatment either absolutely or comparatively. We do not want to leave the impression that analysts have no methods: they do have several, but none are readily accepted by the public.

Second, the ethical context in which treatment for medical problems is undertaken envisions the caregiver, usually a physician, as a source of information, an advisor, and in certain contexts an advocate for the patient. Even more important for our present discussion, the physician serves as advocate for the personal goals and subjective preferences of individual patients, not for classes of patients or for society as a whole. Let us return to our example of total hip replacement for painful arthritis. Given an equal severity of symptoms and an equal operative risk, differences in the *subjective value* attached to the relief of symptoms and the potential for greater physical activity and to the risk of fatality may cause patients with objectively identical conditions to make different decisions. For example, a parent with young children may feel that the risk of an early death, which might leave the children at the mercy of a not very benevolent society, is unacceptable, even though the more likely outcome, the relief of pain, could help him or her care for them.

Guidance from Case Studies

The flowering of laboratory science and biomedical technology in the last fifty years has created an impressive agenda of medical interventions for the evaluator to address. Analysts wish to measure the degree of benefit conferred on patients by individual medical interventions or technologies, and the costs of the resources required to secure those benefits. This agenda still is too long for any small group of analysts to review. In order to make a start on the evaluative task, the authors have adopted a simple strategy for selecting interventions to present in this book. First, we chose interventions whose efficacy is well documented: the health problem addressed must be common, a significant threat to life, function, or comfort, and widespread medical opinion and the technical literature must provide a strong presumption of benefit from use of the intervention.

Second, we chose interventions that may offer lessons about how to improve a national health care system. Now and over the next few years, there may be substantial changes in the structure and financing of our system of health care. For that reason our analysis will pay particular attention to objectives that will continue to be desirable, independent of the details of systemic reforms.

Third, we have confined the analysis to illnesses in the industrialized nations of the world. This choice derives from our greater familiarity with the medical problems of the industrialized nations, and our wish to explore the use of a set of methods to analyze what we think is a broader range of data.

Fourth, other characteristics being equal, we have been swayed in our choice of interventions by the opportunity to diversify the spectrum of policy implications of the analyses.

We chose the method of case studies to describe the salient properties of successful innovations in health care and to identify sources of potential improvement. Our primary concern is the appropriate and productive use of technology assessment in guiding decisions on how to care for patients. One could argue that it is redundant to document medical successes and then to draw out the policy implications of achieving that success. The system brought about the desired result; tinkering might ruin it. Our belief, however, is that even successful policies contain lessons as to how the particular effect might have been achieved more directly, more economically, or yet more successfully.

Themes of the Book

The overarching theme of this book is the importance of technology assessment in achieving success in health care. If we are to have good medical care, we need to know what works, and this cannot be known without systematic technology assessment. The intuitions of physicians and the guesses of biologists are not adequate guides to the best treatments. We break the program for technology assessment into three parts.

First, we want to know how much good is being accomplished by the health care system. To find out, we need to know how many treatments are delivered and what their outcomes and costs have been. Naturally we would also like to know whether they have been appropriately delivered. Thus in order to know how effective treatment has been we must keep careful track of the use of technology. Even further, we should know how successful the treatments have been and how costly both in dollars and in losses when the treatment fails or goes awry, as treatments sometimes do. Our success in this part of the endeavor depends upon our previous success in carrying out evaluations of competitive treatments.

Second, we must carry out careful comparisons of different treatments for the same ailment as a prelude to finding out how well we are doing in particular instances. We want to know which treatments are successful in curing or relieving patients of their infirmities. We need also to know how expensive the treatments are. Discovering what works and at what cost is a major aspect of health technology assessment. When one treatment is more likely to help the patient than another and the costs are comparable, it is easy for us to choose the treatment that is more likely to cure. When treatments are about equally effective and one is less costly, it is easy to choose the less costly one. But a harder problem arises when the treatment most likely to help the patient is only slightly better than its nearest competitor while its cost is very much greater. Most people have not yet made peace with this problem, but we will have to grapple with it as we develop a universal health care system. Of course, a further problem arises when the cost of a treatment is so high that its use, however effective, will threaten to bankrupt the system. The question "How much is too much?" is also one that society has not dealt with systematically so far. To develop our health care system, we must consider both success rates and costs, including properly the benefits society receives when people return to work after an illness and the losses that are associated with long-term care for people who cannot manage on their own.

The third theme of the book deals with the partial success ordinarily achieved by a successful treatment. If a treatment is generally successful, why has it not essentially wiped out the losses attributable to the disease? It is a common experience that a good treatment does not have as much success as it deserves. Part of technology assessment should be to find out why shortfalls occur. The case studies are helpful in illustrating how failures occur and in suggesting improvements in performance that can be identified with specific measures, not only for the example in question but often by extension to other valuable technologies. Thus improving the delivery of successful medical technologies is a third theme of the book.

The Structure of the Book

To identify an innovation as successful, the analyst must demonstrate that the innovation has merit. In Chapter 2 we discuss the features of a technology assessment that establish confidence in the benefits of the innovation and a quantitative understanding of its risks. We then move right on to the case studies, each of which is devoted to the discussion of a particular medical innovation or family of related innovations. The topics are grouped according to the salient policy issue embedded in each technology.

In the final three chapters we turn to the wider application of the principles and methods presented in the case studies. Chapter 17 brings together a series of topics related to technology assessment that cut across the specific innovations described earlier. Chapter 18 deals with the policy implications of the individual cases, which we approach from the broader context of technology assessment in a health care system that is under stress and likely to undergo change. The last chapter offers a series of recommendations whose importance is not likely to be weakened by any upcoming reforms in the health sector.

2

Evaluating Medical Technologies

FREDERICK MOSTELLER AND HOWARD S. FRAZIER

The Lessons of DES

In the 1950s the medical profession had concluded from biological research that the drug diethylstilbestrol (DES) would have a beneficial effect on the course of pregnancy. Some physicians believed that women likely to miscarry or to have premature babies would improve their chances of carrying their babies to full or nearly full term by taking the drug during pregnancy. Many pregnant women were given the drug, even though this hypothesis had not been tested through a randomized, controlled trial, and even though physicians are generally reluctant to expose pregnant women to drugs for fear of damaging the fetus.

Between 1950 and 1954 six clinical studies encouraged the use of diethylstilbestrol, though none of these had controls randomly assigned and none employed double-blinding (we discuss these features of clinical trials later) [1]. Four other studies did have randomized, concurrent controls and blinding, and these disagreed with the first set. They did not report successful use of the drug. Indeed, in this second set of investigations, and in additional studies carried out later, the rates of miscarriages, stillbirths, neonatal death, and premature delivery were not improved in the treated group. On average the outcomes were a bit worse with the treatment, and the number of premature births was definitely higher. Thus the treatment apparently aggravated the very condition it was intended to cure. Nevertheless, the treatment was employed widely over a 30-year period. Goldstein, Sacks, and Chalmers [1, p. 612] call the use of DES "a classic example of the danger of applying pathophysiologic reasoning to therapeutic action without first testing the hypothesis by means of adequately designed trials."

The complaint is not, however, against the original hypothesis, but against the failure to test it before widespread application.

Worse news followed. After a few years vaginal cancer, a rare disease, was increasingly diagnosed in young women. It soon became clear [2] that these women were children of mothers who had had the DES treatment. Very few of the daughters of the treated women developed cancer, though enough did to indicate an association between vaginal cancer and DES. The link was made by an epidemiologic study called a "case-control" study rather than a randomized trial. The study compared women who had the cancer (cases) with women who did not (controls) and found a high rate of DES exposure for the mothers of the first group but not for the mothers of the controls.

Vaginal cancer was not the only adverse effect. Vaginal adenosis appeared at a high rate in the 25-year follow-up of daughters of women who had taken DES. Male offspring of the treated mothers also had a variety of adverse outcomes, though we shall not summarize these.

This chapter introduces a series of ideas, summarized here but developed more fully in later chapters, that must be considered as we evaluate whether medical innovations are beneficial. The history of DES illustrates two important ideas: first, that it is necessary to test a new treatment for both safety and effectiveness; second, that it is also necessary, after a new treatment is adopted, to *continue* careful surveillance of recipients of the treatment in order to detect rare or long-delayed consequences. We discuss a number of further examples of the need for randomized trials and the results of the failure to carry them out (see especially Chapter 14). The need for post-marketing surveillance is emphasized in the chapter on oral contraceptives (Chapter 15), though happily, as illustrated there, sometimes the findings of longer-term studies are welcome instead of tragic.

Randomized, Controlled Trials

Before physicians test a drug on humans, it will already have been examined in many ways. Its chemical structure will have been studied, for example, to see whether it is similar to carcinogenic substances with which physicians and biochemists have had experience and may therefore be likely to cause cancer also. It will likely have been tested for safety on animals that seem to respond to chemicals as humans do. If the drug has been used in humans for some purpose other than the one proposed, that record will have been reviewed. But in spite of all these wise precautions, if the drug is to be used for humans, it must be tried out in humans. Chemical experience and theory and animal experimentation help a lot, but in the end we have to find out how this particular drug works for this particular disease in humans by testing it in a well-designed way that will produce reliable information.

But surely, some will say, if a treatment immediately cures a disease the evidence would be overwhelming. Yes, slam-bang effects occasionally occur; the use of vitamin C for scurvy and antibiotics for certain infections offer marvelous illustrations. Administering these treatments is almost like turning on a switch for a lightbulb. But such innovations are rare. Of the hundreds of new treatments appearing each year, we are fortunate if one or two behave in this way.

If treatments either worked or failed in such a readily recognizable way, much of the problem of evaluation would be quickly solved. Instead, most treatments affect different people in different ways and so the course of

---

James Lind's Famous Experiment

A great killer in naval history and in the annals of far-flung exploratory expeditions was scurvy. During long voyages, scurvy would claim more lives than accidents, warfare, and other diseases. In 1747 the physician James Lind experimented with six dietary additions, each given to two sailors ill from scurvy (Lind, 1753). These included vinegar, seawater, cider, vitriol elixir, oranges and lemons, and a mixture of herbs and drugs. The two sailors receiving the citrus fruit were cured quickly and completely enough that they were able to help nurse the other patients.

A treatment so dramatically successful can be recognized quickly, without large randomized trials. Making sure that the newfound cure is used in practice is sometimes another matter. Although vitamin C was a great success, forty-eight years passed before the British Navy followed up this experiment, done on one of its own ships, and stocked citrus fruits on vessels before long journeys. It took the private sector another seventy years to catch up: only in 1865 did the British Board of Trade decide to require citrus fruit for sailors on long voyages.

Lind, J. 1753 [reprint, 1953]. *A Treatise of the Scurvy.* Edinburgh: University Press.

---

treatment must be viewed as a probabilistic or statistical process. People vary in degree of illness, respond differently to the same medicine, require different amounts of time for treatments to cure them, and some may even find themselves harmed by procedures that do good for others. Consequently, in assessing a new treatment, we need to make sure that we compare its performance in the experimental group with its performance in a control group as similar to it as possible in every way but one: the control group is subjected to a different treatment, such as the treatment that is standard at the time or, when no effective treatment is known, a placebo. Of course, suitable patients participate by their own choice and must give their informed consent.

Matching. In trying to recruit treatment and control groups, one's first thought is to make the groups as alike as possible—same disease, ideally equally severe, same age, same sex, and so on. This matching approach is attractive and is sometimes used to some degree, but it has a weakness. When one tries to match groups on several variables, such as sex (2 groups), age (10 five-year groups), severity of illness (3 groups), and occupation (4 groups), one soon has many categories, here, $2 \times 10 \times 3 \times 4 = 240$. As the number of categories mounts, the chances of finding two or more people matched on all the characteristics sinks. Usually people enlist in an investigation over time, and so it may not be convenient to match them up in this way. Even when we do, there still may be important variables we have not considered. It often happens that after an investigation is well under way one wishes one had matched on a previously overlooked variable, like smoking status.

Thus deep matching is often impractical because the population does not provide enough candidates with matched characteristics. Furthermore, variables not used in matching—possibly unknown variables—may turn out to have an important effect.

Randomization. To get around the problem of the impact of unknown variables, researchers use random numbers to assign patients to the treatment group or the control group. The assignments are made only after enrollment in the trial is firm. This practice avoids a bias that might occur if a physician enrolled patients in anticipation of obtaining a particular treatment for a patient and then withdrew the patient if the treatment was not one the physician preferred. It seems astonishing that random numbers, a device used to create variation, should be a solution to the problem of achieving homogeneity.

Nonrandomized experiments are common. For example, Lind's experiment with adjusting diets to treat scurvy was not randomized. He assigned the sick sailors to the different treatment groups in some way we cannot describe—perhaps "haphazard" would be fair. When we use random numbers, we do something very definite. For example, here is a patch of 25 random numbers:

67089
95037
59459
43279
45285

If we have two treatments we might decide to assign odd numbers to the standard treatment, S, and even numbers to the innovation, I. Since the first number in the table is 6, we would assign the first patient to the innovation I; the second (7) to the standard S; the third (0) to I; the fourth (8) to I; and the fifth (9) to S. Thus we take an active role in making the assignment. In these 25 numbers the split would give 15 S's and 10 I's. Note that a random process may produce uneven groups in the long run. There are methods available to assure that the split is more nearly even, but we shall not pursue this further.

In formal trials the assignment to treatment or control group is usually made from a central authority and information about what treatment goes to the next patient is protected.

The uncertainty of the physician as to the effectiveness of treatments is a key issue in designing a randomized study, for if one were certain which treatment was better, it would be unethical to assign some patients to the inferior treatment simply for the sake of comparison. Furthermore, certainty without good evidence is a hazard—it prevents trials from being carried out just when they are needed.

Historical controls. Sometimes in non-randomized experiments investigators compare the performance of a current group of patients in an institution, such as a hospital or a physician's practice, with patients treated at an earlier time—sometimes under similar conditions, such as the same hospital or the same practice. The earlier patients are called "historical controls." The experience has been that innovative treatments usually look better when we compare current patients with historical controls, sometimes because people are often in better shape than previous generations were. Recall that a major priority of evaluation is ensuring that both the standard treatment and the innovation are applied to equivalent populations of people. When the comparison population is from long ago, and possibly even from a different environment, we cannot expect a fair comparison.

Placebos. The fact that the medical system delivers a treatment often has a powerful effect on both patients and those who care for them. Both groups tend to believe that the treatment will accomplish some good, and this belief is called the "placebo effect." For example, the anesthesiologist Beecher [3] found 32 percent of patients relieved of severe postoperative wound pain by a placebo (such as a sugar pill). And more generally he found coughing, mood changes, angina pectoris, headache, seasickness, anxiety and tension, and even the common cold were reported to have been relieved by a placebo at a rate averaging 35 percent across all these conditions. The substantial size of this effect and its many manifestations in different circumstances encouraged improvements in experimental design that included the use of placebos.

When no treatment, as opposed to "treatment" with a placebo, is given to a control group, the change in the condition of the controls may not be so substantial. In some trials, therefore, a placebo is given to the controls to mimic the experience of the treatment group. It is not always possible to match the treatment by a placebo procedure. For example, if the treatment is a surgical operation, it is regarded now as unethical to carry out a sham operation as a control.

In the early days of clinical trials, a few such shams were carried out and one proved that the real operation was not effective. Angina pectoris is chest pain caused by insufficient blood flow to the heart muscle during exertion. On the basis of experiments related to blood flow, some surgeons conjectured that tying off (ligating) the internal mammary artery would over time improve the blood flow to the heart muscle and relieve the pain [4]. Some other surgeons tried it out on a patient with a substantial history of angina pectoris. The patient improved and was said to be well two years later. After World War II the operation caught on in Europe and the United States, though there was some controversy. Barsamian [4] says the operation became popular because it was safe, simple, applicable to many patients, and seemingly effective. Barsamian notes that the follow-up to an operation where the assessment is difficult and subjective may not be regarded as highly as the opinion of authority. Eventually, though, several studies of the operation were carried out. In two of these [5, 6] a random half of the patients were treated by tying off the artery and the other half were given an incision but were not ligated. Both groups improved with no serious difference in success between the two, though the recipients of the sham operation reported slightly better success. These findings ended the enthusiasm for the operation.

Blinding or masking. Whenever possible the actual treatment delivered— whether a pill is a new drug or the old one or a placebo, for example—is not revealed to the patient or to the personnel who evaluate the outcome of treatments. This concealment is called "blinding" or "masking," and when both patients and evaluators do not know the treatment used the investigation is said to be "double-blind." The problem of identifying a treatment, of course, is the same with evaluators as with patients; they have beliefs or prejudices favoring certain treatments and, being human, their judgments are influenced by them. Again, recall that the outcomes usually are not all-or-none but a matter of degree. Many people would prefer to judge a treatment by the obvious criterion of whether it prevents death, but much of medicine is delivered to improve quality of life or comfort or convenience, and so the life-or-death standard may not be appropriate. Sometimes sophisticated patients, such as nurses, can identify the medication being employed from its taste or from some physical reaction to it. Such problems make concealment more difficult.

Good Research Design

Let us temporarily assume that we have identified all of the relevant types of outcome, good and bad, that we think might occur as a result of a particular treatment for a medical problem. The next task is to make a valid or true measurement of the likelihood that a particular outcome will come to pass. Because the biological characteristics and life histories of human beings are so complex and various, it is not possible to identify simple links of cause and effect to explain many medical outcomes. In- stead, descriptions of possible outcomes are probabilistic. In the course of the last century, enormous advances have been made in the design and development of statistical methods for describing complex populations and events, and in identifying the conditions for gathering the information to which the statistical methods can appropriately be applied. Recently, for example, we have come to appreciate how pervasive and subtle the sources of unconscious bias can be. Because many of the points we make in subsequent chapters are conditioned by methodologic flaws in published studies, we briefly mention here some of the more important attributes of a sound study.

Fulfillment of all criteria noted in this section clearly does not guarantee that the conclusions from a particular study can be believed without further question. Failure of a study to meet one or more of these standards, however, suggests that the conclusions ought to be reviewed with care. In selecting articles for use as case studies, we usually were able to refer to randomized, placebo-controlled, blinded trials (RCT) as the gold standard for measuring the effect of the experimental intervention. We will use the abbreviation RCT as a substitute for the full list of these attributes (described above and below) of a well-designed trial. In addition, a trial, for the sake of validity and efficiency, must begin with an explicit statement of the hypothesis that is to be tested, before the data are examined.

A properly designed study will usually include enough subjects in each group so that a clinically important difference in the response of the treatment and control groups is likely to be detected. Though this feature is a desirable one, it should not be invoked to rule out studies of modest size, because collections of small studies may produce important information if they are well done and carefully combined.

Choosing an adequate sample size helps us address some of the problems created by the probabilistic aspects of an RCT. Consider the example of a trial in which half the patients with a given disease are given one treatment, the rest another treatment. Of course, it can be observed whether one group of patients improved more than the other, but sampling variation— differences between groups that are due simply to chance rather than to the treatment given—must be taken into account. Suppose, for instance, that one treatment does improve half the patients treated when thousands are tested. If we then tested only a hundred patients, would we expect *exactly* fifty of them to improve?

Research in statistics has shown that if we repeated this test of 100 patients many times we would find that in 95 percent of the trials between 40 and 60 patients would improve. Only rarely would exactly 50 of the 100 show improvement, though we would still say that the treatment was beneficial for 50 percent of patients. It is simply a matter of chance variation that in one trial of 100 only 46 patients show improvement while in another trial 53 patients receiving the same treatment do so. When we

compare the outcomes of a treated group and a control group, the difference in counts of successes (improved patients) must be substantial for it
to be compelling evidence that one group did better than the other because
of the treatment and not because of mere chance, which turns out to be
not so mere.

Indeed, if both groups are of size 100, then a difference of 14 successes
(14 more patients improved in one group than in the other) would be
required to meet the usual criterion for recognizing a difference. If in one
treatment group the true probability of success is 0.5 and in the other it
is only 0.4, then the probability that an experiment with two groups of
size 100 will detect which treatment is preferable is about 0.3. (This
probability is called the power of the test and is determined by an equation
too complicated to introduce here.) And so most of the time the difference
in treatment outcomes could not convincingly be argued to be a result of
the difference in treatments. Larger sample sizes are required to increase
the power of the test to detect valuable small differences. When we are
dealing with life and death, small gains like 5 percent or less (such as a
treatment that helps 50 percent of patients versus one that helps 45
percent) may be what we are trying to achieve and retain, and these gains
are even harder to detect convincingly.

Because treatments that produce very large effects are rare, we must
realize that usually relatively small gains arc going to be achieved from the
introduction of new treatments. The important thing is that we have to
detect and document the positive effect of these new treatments. Many
small gains add up to substantial improvements over the years, both for a
specific disease and for other diseases. The progress in the treatment of
childhood cancer has been of that character; many gains of a few percent,
cumulated from many improvements in treatment, have over a few decades
produced valuable improvements in life expectancies for thousands of
young people. An additional way of thinking about these small gains is
that they are being made with respect to many diseases and, since over a
lifetime most of us have many different sicknesses, their total contribution
to life can be substantial.

The size of effect has a substantial impact on the sample size needed to
detect it—the smaller the difference in performance between two treatments, the larger the sample size must be to detect that difference. Consider
again the problem posed by the example noted above: in a small sample
of 100 patients receiving the standard treatment (which improves the

Table 2-1. Sample sizes required for treatment and control groups to detect gains
from an innovation of 2, 5, or 10 percent, given a cure rate in the
control group of 50 percent and a power of 80 percent.

Gain from innovation	Sample size for each group
2%	5,393
5%	859
10%	213

condition of 50 percent of patients), between 40 and 60 of the patients
can be expected to improve. How, then, could we detect a small improvement or loss, of 2, 5, or 10 percent, in the success rate—that is, whether a
new treatment is beneficial to 52 percent of patients, or 55 percent, or 60
percent, instead of only 50 percent?

The evidence usually required to conclude that a small difference in
outcomes in the treatment and control groups is due to the treatment and
not to sampling variation is that the difference be further from 0 (no gain
or loss by the treatment group) than would be found 95 percent of the
time when no gain or loss is actually present. Since we are concerned with
both gains and losses, the 5 percent is the sum of the 2.5 percent of cases
corresponding to an observed gain and 2.5 percent of cases corresponding
to an observed loss. This is the two-sided 5 percent significance level, and
it is used as a standard for reducing the probability that sampling fluctuations will appear to be actual gains or losses due to a new treatment.

In addition, we want power of 80 percent. When there is a difference,
we want a high probability of detecting it convincingly. Thus we not only
want to defend ourselves from being misled by sampling fluctuations (by
meeting the standard of the 5 percent significance level), we want the
samples to be big enough to detect differences of a size we would find
valuable. Naturally it is harder to detect small differences than larger ones,
and that is why larger sample sizes are needed to find them.

Table 2-1 shows that detecting a difference in success rate of 10 percent
at the 5 percent significance level requires treatment and control groups
of size 213. Halving the gain to 5 percent multiplies the required samples
by approximately 4. Reducing the improvement to one-fifth (from 10 to
2 percent) multiplies the number required by about 25. Thus establishing
the existence of small benefits rapidly gets very expensive.

One might argue that even a gain of 0.5 percent (we would need to multiply the 213 by about 400 to get a suitable sample size) would be valuable. If we were able to increase the success rate by 0.5 percent for a disease that killed 400,000 people annually, 2,000 lives would be saved for a time. Physicians would like to save more lives, of course, but the question then would arise whether, among all the ways there might be to save that extra half percent, this is the most effective and economical and sure. Small gains, in addition to being hard to detect, may possibly be more readily achieved by other improvements than the one being considered.

Because we value randomized, controlled trials for determining good treatments, we need to think of ways of getting more of them. But they can be very expensive, especially when large sample sizes are needed. In Chapter 17 we describe a way of organizing hospitals that makes it easier to carry out randomized trials. We also describe there a proposal by Richard Peto to increase the number of large simple trials.

Medical Technology Assessment

The kinds of studies discussed in the first half of this chapter are just one part of medical technology assessment. They answer an important question—Is this particular treatment better than another?—but we have a larger task to consider: the appraisal of medical technologies not only for their efficacy but also for safety, cost-effectiveness, and social and legal desirability. In our view, "technology" refers to more than drugs or devices; we would include intensive care units, surgical operating teams, hospitals, and vaccination programs. Some people would argue that we already know that we need these "technologies," so why do we need technology assessment?

We need technology assessment because medical innovations often fail to deliver the hoped-for benefits. One would like to suppose that any treatment prescribed by physicians had been proved to be successful in coping with the patient's complaint. Although this may be said of many treatments, it is by no means universally true. It is not always possible to *prove* a treatment's worth because the number of treatments and procedures is huge and proof comes at a price. We cannot test every variant of every medical procedure on every patient subgroup. Unfortunately, neither common sense nor sophisticated logic based on biological science can tell us whether a new treatment will do better in practice than the current treatment or even than no treatment. As we will find throughout this book, again and again physicians have been disappointed when well-thought-out innovations in the hands of experts have failed to deliver successful treatments.

A great many methods of evaluating medical technology—standard ways of delivering care as well as new interventions—are available. Table 2-2 lists and comments on a number of these methods. Often more than one approach may be used in a single study because of the variety of purposes a technology assessment may need to serve. In the remainder of this chapter we offer an overview of the research methods and broader issues of concern in the field of medical technology assessment.

Sample surveys. A sample survey obtains data from a sample of the population, ideally from a representative sample—representative in the sense that if a large enough sample is drawn, desired information on properties of the population can be accurately derived. Although a survey seems very different from a good RCT (with randomization, blinding, and so on), it can yield valuable information. Floyd Fowler, John Wennberg, and their colleagues have used this method very successfully in their studies of problems of the prostate [7, 8], for example. One concern to anyone evaluating medical technology is that the literature may be biased, with too many reports from physicians who have had very successful outcomes, and too few reports of failure, being published in medical journals. In a sample survey of surgery for treatment of an enlarged prostate [7], the researchers found that the death rate, the impotence rate, and the incontinence rate were higher than the reports in journals had led them to expect.

The researchers next examined a national sample of Medicare patients treated with radical prostate surgery for cancer of the prostate, which probably represents about two-thirds of all such surgery patients in the United States. They found that fewer than 10 percent reported full sexual function after surgery, over 30 percent reported the need to wear pads to handle wetness, 20 percent required follow-up treatment, and nearly 30 percent needed significant additional treatment for cancer within four years. Thus far there is no strong evidence of benefit from this surgery, and so patients face a dilemma. The substantial side effects raise questions whether cancer patients without significant symptoms should have surgical intervention. In Scandinavia less aggressive treatment is used. In the United States only 3 percent of men die from prostate cancer, though over 30 percent of men over 80 years of age have cancer cells in their prostate

Table 2-2. Methods of technology assessment for evaluating safety and efficacy of treatments, risks, costs, preferences, and extent of current practices.

Method or source	Use	Comment
Randomized clinical trial	To compare performance of different treatments for the same condition	Provides good statistical balance among groups, but eligibility conditions may limit similarity of subjects to the whole population by excluding important classes of patients
Receiver-operating characteristic curve, relating true positive rate to false positive rate	To evaluate diagnostic methods	Recent innovations not yet in wide use
Series of consecutive cases	To give longitudinal summaries of experience with a technology for a physician, hospital, state, or nation	Lack of explicit study design, or protocol, and randomization make findings difficult to interpret or adjust
Case study of a procedure, program, institution, or decision	To determine causes for current state of affairs and reasons for policy decisions, new or old	Conveys complexity of a program or uses of a device; collections of case studies may be of use in studying general issues
Registers and data bases	To maintain systematic records of cases and findings that can be related to other information	When associated with additional information, new research possibilities are created
Sample surveys	To estimate frequency of events in a population, costs, or variability in outcome	Good at representation, usually weak in support of causal arguments
Administrative data	To record information about current usage and its changes, costs, and outcomes	Weak on assessing causation; often difficult to relate outcomes to treatments

Table 2-2.   (continued)

Method or source	Use	Comment
Epidemiologic methods: cohort studies, case-control studies, cross-sectional studies	To support causal analysis in circumstances where experiments may be unethical, impossible, or too time-consuming or expensive	Helpful in studying risk factors and cost-effectiveness
Surveillance	To detect rare or long-delayed side effects of treatments released to market; to monitor performance of preventive methods such as vaccines; to report trends	Current U.S. post-marketing surveillance is relatively weak
Quantitative synthesis methods, including meta-analysis	To combine information from multiple sources in order to summarize effectiveness of different therapies for a common problem	Take advantage, where possible, of previous experience; even when randomized clinical trials are summarized, the synthesis is an observational study, not an experiment; a group of trials contain information not available in single trials
Group judgment methods (Delphi, consensus conferences, etc.), sometimes incorporating literature reviews	To summarize group opinion	Usually do not produce new evidence of safety, efficacy, or cost-effectiveness
Cost-effectiveness and cost-benefit analysis	To evaluate benefits and costs of treatments and procedures relative to one another as well as absolutely (in terms of dollars)	Cost data are difficult to obtain, and therefore charges are often used as a substitute; the approach provides a foundation for attempts to get the most care for a given expenditure

Table 2-2. *(continued)*

Method or source	Use	Comment
Mathematical modeling	To study processes of programs as well as input and outcome, and thus to consider the impact of changes in the process	A major problem is to be sure the model actually describes the steps in the process and is based on realistic assumptions about these steps
Decision analysis	To determine optimal choice	This is a special form of mathematical modeling that takes into account probability of outcomes together with costs and benefits
Examination of social and ethical issues	To consider the impact of procedures and treatments on society generally, both immediately and in the long pull; to consider what is medically appropriate as well as what is legal	Fuchs [9] notes that resources are scarce and that people have different wants, so the economic problem is "to allocate scarce resources so as to best satisfy human wants"

gland. In this instance the sample survey of outcomes of radical surgery raises hard questions about its benefits and shows why a survey can be informative even though no clinical trial has been done.

Cost-benefit and cost-effectiveness analyses. As noted above, technology analysts want to know not only whether a treatment works but also whether it is worth paying for. Two important methods of assessing a treatment's cost, cost-benefit analysis and cost-effectiveness analysis, are widely used. In cost-benefit analysis all the costs of treatment and the benefits from it are weighed in terms of dollars. In cost-effectiveness analysis, costs are compared with years of life gained or lost, sometimes adjusted by a factor intended to account for the quality of life after treatment. Sometimes these methods are used to compare the costs and benefits of different treatments for the same disease, and they also may be used to help decide which treatments should be included in a health care benefits package.

Research synthesis. Among the methods that help us carry out technology assessment is research synthesis. Sometimes these syntheses are called "overviews" and sometimes "meta-analyses." Often in medicine several studies are carried out to examine the "same" problem, as happened in the study of diethylstilbestrol, and they do not always agree in either the qualitative outcome or the quantitative results. Sometimes the treatment given the experimental group is not quite the same in the different investigations, sometimes the populations differ according to age or gender mix, and sometimes the endpoints of the investigations, and the time lapsed between beginning treatment and final data collection, may differ. It may not be possible, then, to compare the results of studies of such different design. Furthermore, in some cases only small studies have been done, for which one must expect large statistical fluctuations.

When comparing or combining several studies, it is not enough just to review their findings by eye. We need to appreciate quantitatively what the data add up to. Specifically, we must take account of the sample sizes of the studies, the equivalences and non-equivalences, and pay attention to the variation in the sizes of effects from one study to another. When we sum up, we want results that can be explained to people, results we can have confidence in.

The general idea of a meta-analysis is to find reports of all the randomized trials and make sure that they are of similar design. Then we want to gather their data systematically and add them up. Why isn't it enough to review just a few studies and see how they come out? One reason is that the person doing the synthesis may have biases in favor of some treatments or in favor of some authors. Therefore, we need protocols for carrying out the investigation to protect the investigators as much as possible from these biases. Recall that the best clinical trials are designed to be operated blindly, to prevent patients or evaluators from knowing what treatment was applied and thus avoid biases. The same idea occurs with respect to research synthesis: following strict protocols helps ensure that the results will be evaluated fairly.

It is astonishing how difficult it is to read research articles and identify carefully just what steps were and were not taken, even when the authors have been thorough in their reports. Readers miss key information, add up the numbers wrongly, and fail to notice factual information. When we collect information from papers for synthesis, we have at least two people extract the same information independently. By getting the analysts to indicate exactly where in the paper they found the required information, we can improve our chances of getting correct results. We find in our own work, for example, that about half the time when two readers disagree, one of them has not found the information and the other one has. If we know where it was found, we can show it to the reader who missed it and settle the conflict quickly.

The first step in research synthesis, as in a clinical trial, is to state the primary question, such as, "Does diethylstilbestrol increase the time until birth?" Then the analyst gathers all the research that deals with the question. We prefer to collect data from randomized trials. Computer searches on what are called data bases (lists of articles) are a good start. Reading abstracts of papers winnows out those studies that do not bear on the original hypothesis. But computer searches rarely find more than about half the available articles. The analyst should also seek out the references in the articles found by the computer and write to scholars indicating what has been found and asking whether other studies should be included. Diligent searching in journals especially likely to publish relevant papers also helps.

Once all possibly relevant studies (often including unpublished studies) are found, the winnowing can begin. Studies in which the treatment was given in different form or dosage, or for too short a time, must be abandoned, for example. Only studies having the conditions meeting criteria established by a protocol are left. Standard statistical methods are then applied to the quantitative results of the studies in the final set. These analyses lead to measures that compare the performance of one treatment to another and also give information about the uncertainty of the difference.

Gathering all the clinical trials in a field, organizing them according to topic, and carrying out research syntheses on each question having adequate randomized clinical trials has been done only for obstetrics, by a team centered at Oxford University [10]. In Chapter 17, we discuss the prospects for carrying out such a program for all of medicine.

Who does technology assessment? The greatest amount of experimentation is sponsored by the pharmaceutical industries [11]. Research in appraising the safety and effectiveness of drugs comes under the approval process of the Food and Drug Administration (FDA). The FDA does not itself carry out these appraisals but takes the information supplied by the manufacturers and decides on the basis of experimentation and outcomes whether drugs can be approved for widespread use.

In addition to the work of this sort done by physicians for the pharmaceutical companies, physicians in hospitals and organizations of physicians in specialties often band together to study treatments for specific diseases [11]. Nearly every physicians' specialty association has a unit devoted to such work. Sometimes the National Institutes of Health (NIH) sponsors investigations as well.

Many organizations do not carry out original investigations but do research synthesis with results from other studies on treatments and procedures related to their specialties. The list of organizations with a unit devoted to either health technology assessment or research synthesis is very large [12].

Within the United States government, the Office of Health Technology Assessment carries out such analyses so as to advise the Health Care Financing Administration whether it is appropriate to reimburse providers for certain treatments. The Office of Medical Applications of Research (OMAR) has a special task; it calls together groups in "consensus conferences" to reach agreement on appropriate treatments. Ordinarily no new data are presented at such conferences. Instead, the speakers review what is known and come to a conclusion on an appropriate treatment in a specific area of medicine. Similarly, the Office of Technology Assessment of the U.S. Congress engages in research synthesis but not original field research.

The Rising Cost of Health Care

The costs of health care and the related matter of access to medical services have become issues of intense concern to consumers, providers, payers, and government. Technology assessment is a means of answering important questions in the current policy debate—Does this treatment work and do its benefits justify its costs?—and as such it may help us rationalize the health care system and perhaps help control costs.

The relation between price and access is conceptually a simple one. Other things equal, an increase in the price of health care will reduce access to it. Over the last 25 years, the unremitting increases in the price of health care have reduced access for some groups in our society; various subsidies have been created by employers and government to facilitate access by others. The price of health care, and the subsidies necessary to make it affordable, are now thought to put an intolerable burden on government, business, or the economy as a whole. Reducing the rate of rise of expenditures for medical services has become a national preoccupation. Because we value much of what we get for those medical prices, it behooves us to try to determine exactly what is causing our health-related expenditures to rise before we impose remedies that may have effects we never intended and do not want. The following is an attempt to identify and briefly describe some of the major influences driving the increased expenditures for health-related services.

Changes in the population served. On average, older people have more medical problems than younger ones and consume more medical services as a result. The U.S. population overall is increasing and, in addition, the fraction of the population that is elderly is increasing. Both factors act to increase the consumption of medical services, and hence the level of health-related expenditures. European countries and Japan have experienced the same demographic changes, but so far they have experienced lower levels of medical inflation.

General price inflation. The floor on which all price inflation stands is the half-century of relatively steady increase in the price of a standard package of goods and services. This price is the measure of the Consumer Price Index (CPI); an increase in the CPI is faced by anyone who consumes goods represented in kind and amount by the contents of the CPI market basket, which is to say almost all of us. For the period from 1981 through 1991, the average annual rate of general price inflation was 4.7 percent.

Medical price inflation. We can evaluate the extent of price inflation seen by groups that are special in one way or another by developing a market basket of goods and services relevant to their needs or activities. For instance, in health-related institutions like hospitals, what we will call the "medical supplies market basket" will have different components, but the weighted price will have the same significance as a measure of the price of hospital inputs as does the CPI for individual consumers. For our reference interval from 1981 through 1991, the price of the medical supplies market basket rose annually at a faster rate, 8.2 percent, than did the price of the CPI market basket, 4.7 percent.

Calculations have often been made to show that a large chunk of the health care bill, perhaps as much as a third, is used to pay for the final stage of illness culminating in death. If we always knew when an illness was terminal, some patients would opt not to spend the money. Society too might demur. But we often do not know, and people do survive for long periods after close calls. However hard-hearted we might be, we cannot expect great savings based on less treatment of terminal illnesses.

The savings at best are likely to be much less than the estimates, perhaps as little as 3 percent, because it is difficult to distinguish the costs of care (tending a patient in a terminal state) from the costs of life-saving (preventing a patient from reaching the terminal state) [13]. It will take great political acumen to confront problems like these and design an acceptable health care system, that is, one that is perceived as nearly fair by nearly everyone.

New medical technology. One characteristic feature of the contemporary health care scene is the frequent introduction of new medical technology: new drugs, medical devices, surgical procedures, even new kinds of organizations or institutions to deliver health-related services. In general, the new medical technology tends to be an add-on to the customary pattern of care, not a substitution of one service or treatment for another. It follows that this new technology is almost certain to increase the cost of care. Estimates of the level of price increase caused by new technologies vary somewhat, but an estimate of about one-third of the overall increase seems reasonable. Many of the newly introduced treatments, when adequately assessed, can be shown to improve the outcomes of care, although the effects only rarely are impressive ones and the price may be large. This association of a modest improvement in results for a high price presents us with an increasingly common dilemma as we confront the fact of limited resources for health care.

One paradox in our enthusiasm for new medical technology is our tendency to underutilize simple, inexpensive, familiar, and effective interventions. An example is our neglect of shatterproof eyeglasses for preventing eye trauma in the workplace while offering expensive treatment after eye trauma occurs.

Inadequately evaluated medical technology. Observers of the health care system in the United States often are surprised to discover that there are traditional and widely accepted treatments that have not been evaluated in sufficient detail for us to be confident that they do more good than harm, or that we can even identify the goods and harms. Grimes [14] reminds the medical profession of these issues in a vigorous discussion with many illustrations. The reasons for this circumstance are many and complex: the technology of evaluation itself is changing; evaluation is expensive (although not as expensive or risky as failing to evaluate!); and ethical considerations, about which responsible people may differ, complicate the evaluation of some treatments.

Overhead costs. The U.S. health care system is notably pluralistic both in its arrangements for delivery of services and in its financing. We call attention here to two examples of diversion of resources from the primary objective of producing and distributing health-related services. The first is our present insistence on recording, pricing, and assigning the prices for services in exquisite detail in order to deal with the large number of different suppliers, providers, and payers. Estimates of the magnitude of this overhead cost vary somewhat; 15–25 percent are illustrative figures. Angell suggests a cost of about 20 percent [15].

Reducing overhead costs, as represented by the bookkeeping and appraisals in our current system of reimbursement, might be achieved in a universal health care system like those of Canada or the United Kingdom, where care is delivered and bills are not sent. Angell suggests this will reduce expenses by 10 percent [15]. Undoubtedly, there will be problems with that or any other system, but any method that could knock out as much as 10 or 15 percent of the total cost of care is worth very serious consideration.

The malpractice system. The problem of malpractice suits and their consequences seems to involve two issues. How do we monitor physicians who are not treating their patients properly? How shall we compensate patients who have suffered from bad practice? We ought to be able to devise something better than the tort system to compensate those harmed. Society still does not have a very good way of detecting and removing physicians whose mode of practice is a danger to the public. As in any professional situation, it is difficult to identify and evict unsatisfactory professionals. Removing them from practice and from their livelihood seems to be such a very severe penalty that it is seldom imposed.

The present malpractice system, based in tort law, does not reliably identify or compensate those injured by negligent practice. It stimulates wasteful use of resources by physicians who perceive a need to protect themselves from litigation. Finally, it has begun to alter the willingness of physicians to enter certain specialties, creating scarcities in certain areas.

Controlling Costs: What Technology Assessment Can Do

All of us involved in the debate over how best to control rising health care costs must realize that we have little control over changes in the population served or general price inflation. We could have modest control over medical price inflation by reducing the rate at which we introduce new technologies or by emphasizing lower-priced technologies. We have found in the study of hypertension (Chapter 10), for example, that trying inexpensive treatments first (if several treatment options are available) and only moving up to more expensive ones when the patient requires them does save money. This idea may have fairly wide applicability.

But the major contributions that technology assessment can make to cost control are the evaluation of new technologies and the comparative analysis of technologies already in use. Providing a treatment, new or old, is wasteful if it doesn't work. We know that good scientists using good science and good logic do not always produce therapies that work. (One famous example is the invention of gastric freezing for treatment of ulcers described in Chapter 14.) And we know that some of our increased costs are due to the introduction of new techniques, which are often expensive. Our concern here is not about the invention or introduction of a new treatment—progress requires this—but about overlooking the need for evaluation. One step toward cost containment would be to make sure that the new treatment is effective *before* it is put into everyday use and covered by insurance. This step is one that the Food and Drug Administration is responsible for in the case of drugs and of some devices. This requirement, also recommended by Grimes, would not necessarily reduce costs, because many new treatments do have value, but it would assure that we get better payback for the money spent on health care [14]. To the objection that delay would impede medical progress, we admit that to some extent it will. But it will also save us from disasters illustrated by the DES story.

After we ensure that wasteful "innovations" are identified before widespread use, we can then think about how to carry out suitable cost-effectiveness analyses of existing, competing treatments. Procedures that most need assessment are those dealing with serious diseases and whose efficacy is not clear to the medical profession. When the choice of procedure to treat a given disease varies a great deal from one region of the country to another or from one physician to another, it is reasonable to ask why. Although a variety of treatment preferences can mean that several equally good treatments are available, it more likely means that the profession is in disagreement about the merits of the procedures. Such situations then demand assessment, especially if the competing treatments are expensive or heroic, such as substantial surgical operations or powerful medications, or if they involve major changes in life style. As an example, John Wennberg and his colleagues used the variation in rate of use of surgical operations from one area to another as a device to identify procedures that needed assessment [16]; for example, they found huge variations in the use of adenoidectomy and tonsillectomy in children among apparently similar regions of Vermont. Another example comes from the work of the Agency for Health Care Policy and Research PORTs, or Patient Outcome Research Teams. PORTs review the procedures associated with several troublesome conditions such as back pain (which hits about 80 percent of people sometime during their lives), acute myocardial infarction (heart attack), prostate problems, cataract management, and several other important conditions.

Our discussion has emphasized the need for safety and efficacy in treatment. Sometimes people feel that technology assessment should have a great deal to say about costs. And they may even expect the assessments to control the costs of the health care system. Costs are of great importance because together with our method of distributing health care they limit what can be delivered. Knowing about costs as well as benefits will help us devise a system that will deliver a market basket of health care that offers as much good for the money budgeted as possible.

At the same time, however, we cannot expect that knowledge of what works and what does not and how much different treatments cost will control the behavior of an industry with hundreds of millions of patients, thousands of physicians and hospitals, and scores of pharmaceutical and insurance companies. Controlling the total cost of the system is a separate enterprise, one that we do not deal with in this book. Society has to consider how much it wants to spend on medical care and figure out what it can afford, and then firmly not buy health care it feels it cannot afford. It must also decide whether people should be allowed to dip into their own funds, if they have them, to purchase extra health care that is not supplied in a national health care plan. Nevertheless, if we are to improve our health care, we are going to have to continue to do research and invent new treatments, even if they cannot all be afforded at a given moment. In order to do this well, we need to take into account what we learn from technology assessment.

In carrying out technology assessments, investigators focus on three main outcomes for the patient: death, morbidity, and quality of life. Inevitably saving lives has been a major focus of medicine, but in developed societies most of medicine is oriented toward reducing morbidity and improving the quality of life of the patient. We go to the physician an average of five times a year, but mainly for relief from pain or discomfort or inconvenience rather than because our lives are threatened. This is because medicine has made great progress in the prevention and cure of the killer infectious diseases that in less developed countries still claim so many lives. The new threat of human immunodeficiency virus (HIV) and acquired immunodeficiency syndrome (AIDS) refocuses attention on death as an outcome and on the costs of morbidity and palliation. The emergence of new diseases and their world-wide distribution reminds the modern world of the threats of previous centuries.

Even though deadly threats continue to require medical management, procedures that get people up and around and make them feel better receive much of our attention in assessing medical technologies. Until recently, except in the field of pain relief, we had few ways to assess improvements in quality of life. In the last few decades, much attention has been given to such assessments, and now measurements of improved function—the ability to care for oneself, work, enjoy one's leisure—and of one's mental state have become available and in many areas standardized [17]. In a few years we will have even better ways of reporting what medical procedures accomplish for quality of life. Just now we have many not quite compatible measures. (We return to this issue in Chapter 17.) These new measures will, we hope, help guide future discussions about how we are to provide and pay for health care in the United States.

Broader Questions about Health Care

Even after randomized clinical trials have shown that a treatment is safe and effective, other considerations may come into play that could rule against the use of an innovation. Apart from the possibility that long-run problems detected in post-marketing surveillance could weigh against the use of a treatment, for example, other considerations could matter as well. Costs could be a major consideration, as when an excellent new treatment costs many times as much as a good treatment already in use. Although the tendency is to want to offer the best treatment available, some costs can be out of sight. Still other possibilities are that something about the treatment is offensive to the law or the customs of the society. We are also familiar with situations in which the society itself is torn by differences in attitudes of subgroups toward certain procedures. Thus safety and efficacy do not always direct practice. To close this introductory part, we briefly mention some of the social, economic, and ethical questions that must be kept in mind as we debate the future of health care in America.

The incentive of returning to work. In evaluating the benefits of treatments, the value to society of returning the patient to work might help justify the costs of the treatment. Returning to work usually is good for both the patient and society, but often the return is impeded by a variety of opposing forces. Employers may not be willing to hire people recovering from certain diseases or continuing in a diseased state, because of anticipated work problems or because of problems with the cost of health insurance. Furthermore, some insurance rules result in perverse incentives, as when patients lose some benefits if they have earnings. This problem has been solved conceptually by proposals for a negative income tax, so that earnings lead to gains not losses, but at a lower rate than 100 percent.

Similarly, often the benefits of retirement or welfare do not encourage the recovering patient to return to work unless the work itself is rewarding. (See also Chapter 7.) Some of these problems are addressable, but they require more integrated arrangements among the various programs of support than the United States is likely to have in the forseeable future. Consequently, return to work is not always a good measure of the effectiveness of treatment.

Problems of equity. When we assess a treatment for its costs, we may approach the problem from a variety of viewpoints. We could evaluate it from the point of view of an individual or from the point of view of society. The individual being treated naturally wants the best treatment money can buy, whereas society, when it pays the bill, might lean more toward the treatment it can afford.

We want the treatment that is most likely to relieve the patient's problem. If several treatments are available and they have differing costs, it may be reasonable to choose a good treatment but not the best, especially when there are large disparities in costs. For example, it is not rare for treatments for the same ailment to vary in costs by factors of ten. If we choose to give up a little efficacy, many more people can be treated for the same total cost, and the health budget can be distributed more equitably.

To what diseases should society respond, and with what treatments, if it could deliver an ideal health care package? Ideally, of course, it would offer everything and the best, but economics teaches us that society cannot afford to provide unrestricted amounts of free goods. The demands quickly outrun the supply. The wonderful inventions in medicine are often very expensive, at least when they first appear (and often for a long time thereafter!). Examples are the newer antibiotics ("third-generation" cephalosporins), diagnostic imaging (such as computed tomography scans and magnetic resonance imaging), and tissue plasminogen activator for dissolving clots. With the elaborate work done in robotics, we can anticipate prosthetics that will be astoundingly clever but also stunningly expensive. Society cannot afford to provide the best of these devices to everyone who could use one. In another field, childless couples may wish to try to use some of the newer mechanisms for reproduction, which are expensive and often require many attempts.

In trying to treat people equitably with limited resources, inevitably choices have to be made. The question arises how large the budget should be. Once that is determined, we have to rank-order the treatments that will be delivered. Most attempts to do this have led to difficulties.

If society decides not to pay for procedures that cost more than a given amount for each year of life gained, then people needing such procedures are the ones not served. If we give a priority order to disease-procedure pairs and decide to pay for all pairs in order until the money runs out, then the people at the bottom of the list are discriminated against.

The main point to note here is that ultimately there must be rationing, because no country can pay for all the beneficial treatments that could, in principle, be provided. When the decisions about allocations are made, some groups will be discriminated against. Society needs some good ways of deciding how much health care it can provide and how it wants to distribute these benefits among its members.

As we make these choices, there are special traps that we want to avoid. For example, one proposal is to evaluate a procedure according to the cost of the additional quality-adjusted life-years it provides. In the current debate over lifesaving procedures, people often think that a year of life for a severely handicapped person may not be as valuable as the year for someone not so impaired. Thus approaches that depend on judgments about quality of life tend to bias against providing treatments for special groups. The members of some of these groups do not agree with the evaluations of others about the benefits of their lives. But those who propose making these "quality-of-life" adjustments ordinarily use the judgment of the whole population rather than the judgments of the afflicted, and this may lead to discrimination.

We as a society need to develop our political and quantitative skills to resolve the problems of equity and values posed by rationing questions. We cannot eliminate the element of discrimination that rationing procedures entail, but we might be able to develop a process regarded as fair and acceptable by nearly everyone. As we do so, we will have to confront a major difficulty, and that is our own compassion. Ultimately, we will have to face the problem that special compassion for one person may lead to lack of compassion for other equally deserving but less publicized or less appealing patients.

PART B

Physician Performance

We begin with a set of three case studies that examine important medical innovations whose full exploitation for the good of patients depends on our ability to improve the performance of practitioners. The first innovation, a surgical procedure for removing the gallbladder, involves the introduction of a complex new technology. The new procedure requires a new set of skills on the part of the surgeons, who require training and practice. Is the new treatment a real improvement over the old one? Who should be responsible for the management, including the pricing, of the new technology and the training it requires? The second case also involves a new technology—the use of lasers to alleviate the damage done to the retina by diabetes—but here the issue is ensuring that patients who would benefit from the treatment are identified and treated. If we find that primary caregivers too often overlook the retinal damage in its early stages, when treatment would be most effective, should expensive, large-scale screening programs be instituted? Our third case does *not* involve a high-tech innovation. Several alternatives are available for the treatment of depression, yet many depressive individuals remain untreated. In this case what seems to be needed is to educate physicians about these alternatives and to evaluate their comparative advantages and disadvantages. We can improve physician performance if we can present caregivers with convincing evidence concerning the benefits of treatment.

3

Laparoscopic Cholecystectomy for Gallstones

LEON D. GOLDMAN

The Trouble with Gallstones . . .

Gallstones—hard masses made up of varying amounts of cholesterol crystals, bile pigments, calcium, and sometimes bacteria—may be found in the gallbladders of 15 million people in the United States. Formed by a complex process influenced by the chemical and physical constituents of bile and the gallbladder, they cause symptoms of varying severity in about 10–30 percent of people who have them. The most common symptom is a steady pain located in the right upper or central upper part of the abdomen lasting a few minutes to hours, usually at night. The pain is often recurrent and at times associated with bloating, belching, nausea, and vomiting.

At a minimum these episodes, known as biliary colic, cause mild discomfort and are an annoyance. At worst, they cause intense pain, require hospitalization, intravenous fluid therapy, and pain relief by narcotics. Patients having symptoms, no matter how mild, are at risk for developing more dangerous complications, such as acute cholecystitis (a severe acute infection of the gallbladder), empyema of the gallbladder (pus in the gallbladder), cholecystoenteric fistula (an abnormal connection from the gallbladder to the intestine), or bile-duct stones with cholangitis (a severe infection of the bile ducts in the liver). All of these conditions are life-threatening and may require emergency surgery. Of patients who develop mild or nonspecific symptoms, about 6 percent per year will have recurrent symptoms over time, and about 1 percent per year will develop complications such as acute cholecystitis.

The economic impact of gallbladder disease is substantial. Of the 15 million people in the United States who have gallstones, 10–30 percent will have symptoms of varying severity. Of these 1.5 to 4.5 million people, one-half million undergo surgery for treatment and an unknown portion undergo alternative therapies (which will be discussed below). The remainder do nothing and accept minimal symptoms or suffer in silence until a major problem forces them to do something. It is estimated that the direct costs related to gallbladder disease in the United States are about $5 billion annually.

Treatment

A decision to treat a patient depends on making the diagnosis. In the past, the diagnosis of gallstones was made only after a patient came to the doctor with symptoms of biliary colic. These symptoms and their associated disability provided the indications for treating these patients. Today the decision is more complex. Current diagnostic techniques for other problems may reveal the presence of gallstones, making the gallstones an incidental finding. Treatment of these patients would be a prophylactic measure against the risk of developing a complication. Current opinion holds that patients who have no symptoms from their gallstones or who have had only one minor attack of pain are at little risk of developing a serious complication if they are watched and receive no therapy until they develop further symptoms [1].

Therapy for gallstones is reserved for those patients who have symptoms or complications from their gallstones, or for those who are at great risk of developing an acute life-threatening complication even though they are not yet symptomatic. There is debate over which patients fall into the latter category. For example, the "at-risk" category may include patients with diabetes and patients with a single large stone over 3 centimeters in diameter (because of the association of such stones with gallbladder cancer).

Open cholecystectomy. In an ideal world, therapy would alleviate symptoms, prevent complications, and prevent recurrence of the disease, and it would do so at minimal risk. Cholecystectomy, the surgical removal of the gallbladder, is the closest we come today to this ideal. By removing the gallbladder and the stones within it, the symptoms are alleviated, recurrence of stones is prevented (no gallbladder, no gallbladder stones), and future complications are avoided. Removal of the gallbladder through an open incision into the abdominal cavity (open cholecystectomy, or, for

Table 3-1. Mortality, morbidity, and bile-duct injury in five series of patients undergoing open cholecystectomy.

Series	Study years	No. of patients	Mortality (%)	Morbidity (%)	Bile-duct injury (%)
Ganey et al. [2]	1978–83	1,035	0.5	3.5	NR
Gilliland et al. [3]	1982–87	671	0	4.5	0.4
Habib et al. [4]	1976–81	1,000	1.2	6.3	0.4
Herzog et al. [5]	1984–90	1,631	0.8	NR	NR
McSherry [6]	1932–84	10,749	0.56	NR	NR

NR = Not reported.

brevity, "open chole") has a long and successful history. It was first performed in 1882 and has been performed hundreds of thousands of times over the intervening years.

The operation provides relief of pain in 99 percent of patients who present with biliary colic, and relief of associated dyspeptic symptoms, such as nausea, belching, and heartburn, in 88 percent. Data in the literature attest to its safety, as can be seen in the five studies in Table 3-1 [2–6]. Mortality rates are low. The largest series of data collected over the longest time is from McSherry, who reported the experience at Presbyterian Hospital in New York City over a period of fifty years [6]. Over 10,000 patients were reviewed. Overall mortality was 0.56 percent. Broken down by age, the rates were 0.4 percent mortality for patients younger than 50, 1.5 percent for patients aged 50–64 years, and 4.5 percent for those aged 65 years and older. Another study, done by Herzog and colleagues on 1631 operations from 1984 to 1990, noted a 0.18 percent mortality overall [5]. Gilliland and Traverso, reporting on elective open cholecystectomies done between 1982 and 1987, found a mortality rate of 0 percent in a series of 671 patients [3].

Morbidity rates following the operation are also low, ranging from 3.5 to 6.3 percent, as shown in Table 3-1 [2–4]. The complications referred to here include minor ones, such as simple wound infections, the need for urinary catheters postoperatively, or vein irritation from an intravenous catheter, and major ones, such as pneumonia, renal failure, or injury to the bile ducts. The morbidity rate varies with patient characteristics; an older patient with heart disease, for example, is more likely to experience complications than a younger and healthier one. Incisional pain and its effects have not been looked at in the past, being regarded as an inevitable consequence of surgery (see Chapter 8). Bile-duct injuries have been studied specifically because they represent a complication unique to biliary surgery and may lead to multiple operations and significant disability. As noted in Table 3-1, bile-duct injury rates are low (approximately 0.4 percent). Because of its effectiveness, safety, and long history, open chole has become the standard to which all other therapies for gallstones are compared (the "gold standard").

Alternative therapies. Although open chole is safe and effective, it is associated with pain and disability. Up to 50 percent of patients complain of pain at the incision site for 1–2 years after surgery [7]. Surgery and then convalescence interfere with daily activities and cause economic losses for both the patient and society. Following open cholecystectomy, up to two-thirds of patients spend more than six weeks away from work [7]. For these reasons, people have sought alternative, nonsurgical therapies for gallstones. The two most notable have been dissolution therapy and extra-corporeal shock-wave lithotripsy (ESWL).

With dissolution therapy the patient takes medication that alters the composition of bile so that the stone dissolves. Currently this is accomplished with ursodeoxycholic acid, a bile salt. The agent works only for stones made of cholesterol, however. As a result it is effective in only about 38 percent of patients overall, and the stones reform in about 10 percent of patients per year. ESWL shatters the stone with shock waves; patients then are treated with ursodeoxycholic acid to dissolve those fragments that do not pass spontaneously. Less than 15 percent of patients with stones are candidates for this therapy, and recurrence rates are similar to those for dissolution therapy [7].

Other therapies have been tried but they are more invasive than ESWL and dissolution therapy and do not permanently rid the patient of gall-stones.

Laparoscopic cholecystectomy. The search continued for a therapy that was as safe and effective as open cholecystectomy without the associated pain and disability. In 1989 a newly introduced procedure, laparoscopic cholecystectomy ("lap chole"), seemed to accomplish these objectives. Since it removed the gallbladder, everyone assumed it would be as effective as open chole. In addition, early reports suggested that the resulting pain and disability were minimal.

Lap chole is performed by inflating the abdominal cavity with carbon dioxide gas and then inserting four tubes (called "trocars") through the abdominal wall. A telescope attached to a video camera—the laparoscope—is placed through one of the trocars; this allows the operating team to see the progress of the operation. The operating instruments are introduced through the other trocars and the gallbladder is dissected from its usual site under the liver and removed through one of the trocars.

From the time it was first described in 1989, lap chole spread through the U.S. surgical community faster than any previous surgical technology. Educational courses, many without controls on their quality, sprang up everywhere, and surgeons flocked to learn this new technique. By 1990, the *New York Times* reported that over 5,000 surgeons had taken such courses [8]. The lay press portrayed the procedure as one of the great advances of our time. The public, mesmerized by the prospect of a painless way to remove gallbladders, among other influences, fueled the demand for the procedure. The medical-supply industry responded with more courses and better instruments. The academic community was slow to adopt the procedure because few critical data about its value were available, but it flourished in other settings. By 1992, it was estimated that 15,000 surgeons had received some training, and 80 percent of cholecystectomies were being done by this technique [9].

Because of the intense public demand for this procedure, efforts to mount a randomized, controlled trial comparing lap chole and open chole were unsuccessful. Patients simply were unwilling to participate if there was a chance they would be randomly selected for open chole, the standard operation. Early studies were reviews of the personal experiences of surgeons already enthusiastic about the procedure and eager to see it accepted. Results of these early studies were also skewed by the inexperience of the surgeons. The learning phase for the procedure is pronounced, and early reports have higher complication rates than later reports [10]. Bile-duct injury rates of around 2 percent, five times higher than those of open chole, were being reported in early studies. It was these early results that led many to question whether lap chole should replace open chole, as it appeared to be doing.

With time, more experience was obtained and careful reviews and large prospective series were collected. Table 3-2, which shows four series of data collected by surgeons, reflects the outcomes of surgeons with experience [11–14]. Lap chole can be done safely. Mortality rates range from 0 to 0.3

Table 3-2. Outcomes of laparoscopic cholecystectomy in four series of patients.

Series	No. of patients	Mortality (%)	Morbidity (%) Major	Morbidity (%) Minor	Bile-duct injury (%)	LOS[a] (days)	Work[b] (days)
Meyers [11]	1,518	0.07	1.5	3.6	0.5	1.2	NR
Soper et al. [12]	647	0.0	1.6	2.1	0.2	1.1	8.4
Bailey et al. [13]	375	0.3	0.6	2.9	NR	1.3	7
Graves et al. [14]	304	0.0	0.7	1.3	0.3	NR	7.35

a. Average length of hospital stay in days.
b. Average number of days to return to work.
NR = Not reported.

percent. Further, rates of major and minor morbidity are between 2.0 and 5.1 percent. In experienced hands, ductal injury rates are 0.2 to 0.5 percent, comparable to those found after open chole.

Lap chole does have problems that are unique to the technique. There are injuries related to trocar placement. There are also physiologic changes related to filling the abdominal cavity with carbon dioxide gas under pressure. Increases in the level of carbon dioxide in the blood increases the acidity of the blood as well as blood pressure. These changes can have detrimental effects on patients with pre-existing cardiopulmonary disease [15].

Lap chole also has benefits. Patients need smaller amounts of injected narcotics for pain relief after lap chole and start using oral medication very much sooner. Patients also have been shown to have significantly improved pulmonary function in the immediate postoperative period compared with those undergoing open chole. This is all taken as an indication that patients undergoing lap chole have significantly less pain than patients undergoing the open operation.

Time in hospital and time to return to normal activity are less for the laparoscopic procedure: approximately 1.2 days versus 8.2 days for open cholecystectomy. Bailey and colleagues reported that patients undergoing lap chole returned to normal activity on average in 7 days, whereas those undergoing open chole did not return to normal activity for 35 days [13]. The long convalescence required by open chole, cited above [7], reinforces the point about the economic losses associated with the traditional treatment.

The Cost of Care

The effects of the diffusion of lap chole on financial resources are mixed, at least in part because of the lack of a close relationship between the prices of medical services and their true or resource costs. Given the reduction in the length of hospital stay for lap chole, it is reasonable to expect that the true costs of lap chole would be lower than those for open chole, although the ratio of the hospital-related charges might not reflect this at a particular time in a particular institution. In general, the reported experience indicates some savings attributable to lap chole, but the savings is reduced by the expense of the new equipment required, much of which is disposable.

Potential cost savings due to the substitution of lap chole for open chole are reduced by another circumstance: the rise in the fees of surgeons and anesthetists for performing the procedure. For 1990, South Carolina Blue Cross and Blue Shield reported that surgical fees for lap chole were 55 percent higher than for open chole and that anesthetists' fees were increased by 34 percent [16]. Surgeons have argued that the fees are higher for lap chole because it is a more advanced technique requiring special skills and training, and therefore deserving of higher compensation. Although this was true in the first few years, it may not be the case as lap chole becomes more commonplace and a routine part of the training of all surgical residents. The argument also raises the important policy issue of whether surgical fees should be reevaluated on a regular basis, especially for new procedures. As a procedure becomes more routine and efficiently done, should it be compensated at the same level that it commanded when it was first introduced? We return to this issue below.

As for the anesthetists' fees, these are related to time in the operating room and in 1990 probably reflected the increased operating times associated with lap chole early in a surgeon's experience.

The explosion of new equipment is another factor whose impact on the costs of lap chole is uncertain. Open cholecystectomy is performed with routine surgical instruments, almost all of which are reusable. Laparoscopic cholecystectomy requires special instrumentation, which is quite expensive: not only the video systems and their associated telescopes and cameras, but also special systems to deliver carbon dioxide gas and entirely new operating instruments, such as special scissors, dissectors, and cautery units. Some of the surgical instruments are not reusable. Voyles and colleagues have argued that with careful management, including refraining from using disposable items, the costs of lap chole can be kept down [17]. However, no satisfactory analysis has been done that includes the actual charges for disposable items and factors in costs such as cleaning and repairing reusable instruments.

In summary, lap chole is a safe and effective treatment in trained hands. It offers patients an improved cosmetic result, less pain, and faster return to home and normal activity than does open chole. It does so without measurably increasing the morbidity and mortality of the treatment, once the initial learning phase of the surgeon is passed. Some have suggested that lap chole should become the new "gold standard" of treatments for removal of the gallbladder, the one to which alternative methods would be compared in future.

Policy Issues

The introduction of laparoscopic surgery, unlike most other changes in surgery and medicine, was not an incremental or evolutionary development. It is not an exaggeration to say that it was a discontinuity in technique. Evaluation of the evidence for the safety and effectiveness of new medical devices before their introduction to the market, such as those instruments required for laparoscopic surgery, is the responsibility of the Food and Drug Administration (FDA). Once the devices are deemed safe and effective, the second essential step in dissemination of a safe and effective surgical procedure is the training and then the credentialling of the practitioners who will perform the operation. The authority of the FDA is a highly centralized one. In contrast, the credentialling of practitioners is highly dispersed, typically being the responsibility of the Chief of Surgery in each individual hospital.

The novelty of lap chole and the speed with which interest in it increased overburdened the credentialling function. Initially, there was insufficient expertise and time to design training programs, formulate standards for credentialling, and accumulate adequate experience with both. The result was an impression of unevenness in the quality of performance of practitioners, particularly in the early phases of diffusion of lap chole.

One lesson to be learned from the history of lap chole is that patients might have been better served if the relevant subspecialty professional societies had been more aggressive in designing and overseeing training programs, setting criteria, and developing credentialling standards in order to assist the many Chiefs of Surgery ensure safe practices. The cost of increasing controls over the introduction of a new procedure, of course, is slower diffusion of the procedure, and, if the innovation is ultimately beneficial, the delayed delivery of those benefits to the public. As in other areas of medicine, there is a tension between slowing diffusion of an innovation in the interests of safety and temporary loss of access to a desirable treatment. Appropriate evaluation of new treatments is crucial to the proper workings of a system of health care, but it takes time.

The technical novelty of lap chole meant that almost all practitioners started from scratch in learning to perform the procedure. In consequence, the time required to carry out the lap chole operation tended to be longer than that required for open chole, at least early on. The greater operating time, plus the need for an indeterminate period of special training, was used to justify an increase in the fees for cholecystectomy. With experience, the length of time to perform a lap chole could be expected to fall, and the cost of the special training would be amortized over many more operations. Both of these circumstances would be expected to result in a decrease in the average professional fees for lap chole, but the fees remain at their initial level. Periodic review of professional fees, particularly for new services for which experience will quickly bring increased proficiency and reduced effort, seems worth exploring.

Finally, surgical innovations like lap chole require the training of practitioners if society is to reap the benefits of the new procedure. In this case, the training costs are high. One must not only have expensive equipment but also laboratory space, an animal facility, and appropriate faculty. Industry provides a significant part of the funding for these training programs, with much of the remainder coming from fees charged to the physicians being trained. In both cases, the costs ultimately are incorporated into the charges for the medical service. Conflicts of interest may arise if the medical-device industry controls the content of training programs that influence how the industry's products are used, and these conflicts should be identified as a matter of public policy. In the case of drugs, we have decided that there is a societal interest in appropriate evaluation and use of medications, and so we have injected a neutral expert, the FDA, into the decision-making process. At present, the introduction and dissemination of new surgical procedures do not require input from the public or a neutral expert regarding either evaluation or use. Whether we wish to preserve this difference in the handling of new drugs and new surgical procedures is a topic that merits explicit discussion.

Editors' Note

In contrast to drugs and new medical devices, which are reviewed and approved for use by the federal Food and Drug Administration, operations do not undergo any central review. Responsibility for judging the competence of surgeons to perform them is vested in the Chief of Surgery of each individual hospital. When the adoption of some novel technology is proceeding too rapidly for proper evaluation, the relevant medical specialty societies should be asked to join the process of formulating standards, sponsoring training programs, and credentialling surgeons.

In the short term, the sponsorship, direction, and financial support of training by manufacturers will still be required, despite what may be a significant conflict of interest. Pending the assumption of these responsibilities by academic programs, the surgical leadership should move to take over direction of the training as well as the credentialling of laparascopic surgeons.

Although it may be reasonable to set generous surgical fees during the adoption phase of a new procedure, later savings in time, effort, or complexity should be documented through periodic review and should result in a downward revision of the fee schedule.

Finally, the stresses of rapid adoption of this novel surgical technique highlight the importance of evaluating the risks and benefits of new operations.

4

Preserving Vision in Diabetic Retinopathy: The Impact of Laser Treatment

MICHAEL R. ALBERT AND DANIEL M. ALBERT

Diabetes and the Eye

Diabetes mellitus has been known for centuries. It was recognized by Hippocrates, the father of medicine, who lived about 400 B.C. Prior to the discovery of insulin in 1921, however, the diagnosis of diabetes in children or young adults was tantamount to a death sentence. Even with the development of near-starvation diets in the early part of the twentieth century, a diabetic could not hope to survive for many years, and the quality of life for a sufferer was grim. When two Canadians, F. G. Banting and C. H. Best, discovered insulin in 1921, they opened up a new world for diabetic patients. In patients with longstanding diabetes, however, even when the disease is well controlled, health problems develop. Among the most severe of these are changes in the eyes and in the kidneys.

Diabetes is now known to be caused by the body's inability to produce the hormone insulin or to use effectively the insulin supply it has. Insulin, which is produced in the pancreas and secreted into the blood and distributed throughout the body, regulates a complicated series of biochemical reactions primarily involving glucose. When insulin is lacking or cannot be used effectively, glucose is not transferred to the cells and broken down for energy. This leads to elevated glucose levels in the blood and, consequently, in the urine.

Twelve million people in the United States have the disease diabetes mellitus. There are two main types: Type I, insulin-dependent (previously called juvenile-onset) diabetes, and Type II, non-insulin-dependent (previously called adult-onset) diabetes. Type I usually affects children and young adults below the age of 35. The onset is abrupt and the pancreas produces little or no insulin. The symptoms include excessive thirst and appetite and excessive urination. Although this is the picture usually associated in the public's mind with diabetes, Type I accounts for only 10–15 percent of all cases. In Type II, or non-insulin-dependent, diabetes, the pancreas may produce insulin, but in varying amounts. Unfortunately, the body cannot make efficient use of the available insulin. This type of diabetes, whose onset is gradual, usually affects patients over 35 years of age, and patients often have no symptoms. Among diabetics, 85–90 percent have the Type II variety.

Patients with Type I diabetes usually require regular injections of insulin to compensate for the lack of this hormone. Patients with Type II diabetes may be treated with insulin but may not require it, or their condition may be managed with oral drugs capable of increasing insulin output (antihyperglycemic medications). A discussion of the causes of diabetes is beyond the scope of this chapter.

Most diabetics eventually develop a related disease of the retina known as diabetic retinopathy, or damage to the retina caused by small aneurysms and hemorrhages or scarring of the blood vessels. The retina is the light-sensitive layer of the eye and has been likened to the film of a camera. The risk of developing diabetic retinopathy increases with increasing duration of diabetes. While the cause of the retinopathy is controversial, the majority of investigators believe it is the result of elevated blood glucose, or hyperglycemia. Since patients who are using insulin still develop retinopathy, it has been concluded that insulin replacement does not control all of the metabolic abnormalities caused by the disease. At this writing (1994), a large-scale study known as the Diabetes Control and Complication Trial is being carried out throughout the United States and Canada under the sponsorship of the National Institute of Diabetes, Digestive Diseases, and Kidney Diseases. Its purpose is to compare patients who maintain "tight" blood-glucose control with those who maintain "standard" control. The results should help clarify how large a role hyperglycemia plays in the development of diabetic retinopathy.

Both the doctor who looks in the living eye of the diabetic patient with the ophthalmoscope and the pathologist who examines the eye with the microscope categorize the retinal changes in two major subgroups. The milder types of changes are called *background* or *non-proliferative retinopathy*. The more severe changes, which threaten vision, are termed *proliferative retinopathy*.

Background retinopathy occurs when abnormal capillary dilatations, or *microaneuryms*, rupture blood vessels, allowing serum or blood to leak and form *exudates* or *hemorrhages*. In addition, the abnormal vessels develop clots within them and become occluded. The fine blood vessels of the retina become increasingly porous, and plasma is deposited within the wall of the eye. These nonproliferative changes do not lead to significant visual loss unless they are accompanied by swelling of the portion of the retina most critical for acute vision (the *macula*). If macular swelling (edema) occurs, the patient will notice a decrease in vision.

Proliferative retinopathy results from the lack of oxygen and nutrients in the retina. At this stage new vessels extend from the large veins of the retina. Ironically, the new vessels, which in other organs under similar circumstances are an aid to repair and recovery, damage the retina. Incompletely formed and poorly supported by cells and tissue, the new vessels initially grow in the space between the retina and the vitreous, the gel that fills the back of the eye. Eventually, these vessels invade the gel. Bleeding is common at this stage and may result in temporary loss of vision. Unless treatment is undertaken, a fibrous component or scar-like tissue develops. In many cases this "scar" contracts and detaches the retina from the fibrous wall of the eye, causing permanent blindness.

Prevalence of Diabetic Retinopathy

It is estimated that at the time of clinical diagnosis of diabetes mellitus, retinopathy is present in less than 1 percent of patients under 40 years of age. In patients over the age of 60 years, however, clinical retinal changes may be present in 5–20 percent of affected patients. In all age groups, the frequency of retinopathy rises with increasing duration of diabetes. Among patients who have had diabetes for 10–15 years, 50 percent have diabetic retinopathy. After 20–25 years of diabetes, 80 percent or more have retinopathy.

In patients with Type II diabetes, the retinal changes are usually mild at first but may progress to an advanced stage. Among Type I diabetics, 75 percent will develop proliferative retinopathy within 20 years of onset of the disease.

What impact does diabetes have in the United States? This disease is the principal cause of blindness in working-age Americans, and it accounts for at least 12 percent of the new cases of blindness each year in the United States. On the basis of data from an epidemiologic study, it is estimated that 700,000 Americans have proliferative retinopathy and that 65,000 new cases occur annually. Half a million patients have edema (swelling) of the critical macular area of the retina because of diabetic retinopathy, with impairment of vision. Approximately 75,000 Americans develop macular edema each year. Most sobering of all, approximately *8,000 Americans develop blindness annually* as a result of the complications of diabetes.

Many ophthalmologists and internists believe that diabetic patients who have achieved satisfactory control of their disease through careful diet, oral medications, or insulin treatments have a lower frequency of retinopathy than those whose diabetes remains under poor control. It must be acknowledged, however, that it is difficult to evaluate and correlate the control of diabetes with the development of retinal changes. In some cases retinopathy progresses in the face of careful control and, conversely, in others, when the disease is not well managed, retinopathy is mild and only slowly progressive. The ability of careful control to prevent progressive diabetic retinopathy should become clearer with the completion of the large and elaborately controlled Diabetes Control and Complication Trial previously mentioned.

Management of the Effects of Diabetes

Now that diabetics live longer because of insulin treatment, diabetic retinopathy has become increasingly frequent. In fact, over the course of a few decades, what had once been an uncommon finding became a leading cause of blindness and visual disability throughout the world. To combat this complication, a number of treatments were tried.

One of the most drastic treatments for diabetic retinopathy was *ablation or eradication of the pituitary.* It was demonstrated in the 1930s that destruction of the pituitary improved experimental pancreatic diabetes. A number of patients with diabetic retinopathy were subsequently subjected to surgical removal or destruction of the pituitary gland or to transection of the pituitary stalk. In other patients the pituitary was destroyed by radiation or by the insertion of radioactive implants. This treatment was undertaken only in the most severe and advanced cases and improvement of the diabetic retinopathy was reported. The high mortality rate and hormonal complications of pituitary destruction raised lasting questions about its legitimacy as a method of treatment, and pituitary ablation has since been discarded.

Insulin. The injection of insulin, the hormone that is essential for the proper use and storage of ingested sugar in the body, is the treatment for diabetes most familiar to the public. The insulin used by diabetics is prepared from pancreatic tissues of cattle or pigs or may be synthesized using molecular genetic techniques. Short-acting, intermediate, or long-acting insulins are available. A major drawback of insulin is that it is administered only by injection, and the insulin dosage must be balanced against diet and exercise. If the blood sugar falls abnormally low (a condition known as hypoglycemia) because of excessive insulin dosage, the resulting "insulin reaction" may be dangerous to patients.

As an alternative to insulin, oral hypoglycemic drugs, which act by stimulating the pancreas, are sometimes prescribed in the treatment of diabetes. These are particularly useful in treatment of the mild form of diabetes found in patients over the age of 40.

Pancreas transplants. A strategy for restoring natural secretion of insulin in the diabetic is *pancreatic transplantation.* Either an entire pancreas is taken from a cadaver, or a portion of pancreas is taken from a living donor, for transplantation. The results are somewhat controversial. Because of the high rejection rates and the side effects of anti-rejection drugs, this operation has had very limited use. A more promising avenue of research appears to be the transplantation of clusters of the particular cell type that makes insulin, the beta cell, taken from human fetal tissue or other species. Such cells have been experimentally transplanted with success from one species of animal to another.

Introduction of New Technology:
The Lightcoagulator and Lasers

The use of light in the therapy of retinal diseases was first tried by Meyer-Schwickerath, who in 1949 attempted to focus sunlight in order to produce a burn in the retina to destroy the defective vessels and diminish leakage. This pioneer in the use of light coagulation five years later reported the more practical and simpler technique of using a bright source of light from a xenon arc. In 1959 Meyer-Schwickerath first reported on the use of light coagulation in the treatment of diabetic retinopathy.

Prior to the introduction of the laser, the light coagulator played an important role in the treatment of retinal disease. It was, however, a large and awkward instrument to use, and it made relatively large burns in the retina.

In 1960 the first laser was built in the United States. The laser generates and amplifies a high-intensity, highly monochromatic, and directional (coherent) light. The word *laser* is an acronym for *Light Amplification by Stimulated Emission of Radiation*. By 1961 lasers were being used in medicine, and the most important clinical use has been the treatment of diseased retinas. The energy from a laser focused on a very small spot on the retina could destroy closed vessels and seal weak vessels; it could also produce "spot welds," or focal coagulation, and direct the formation of scar tissue to re-attach a separated or detached retina.

It was also in the 1960s that some ophthalmologists attempted to treat the new vessels of diabetic retinopathy with xenon-arc photocoagulation [1]. Heat was produced when the bright light generated by the xenon arc was absorbed by the pigmented layer of the retina or by hemorrhages on or within the retina. The result was large, slowly formed, moderately intense burns within the eye which caused the new vessels to narrow and the blood flow within them to slow. However, the xenon-arc photocoagulator could not concentrate enough energy in a short enough time to close off or destroy these vessels in the vitreous gel or on the optic disk. Other ophthalmologists attempted treatment with a more powerful source of energy, the red beam of the ruby laser or the blue-green beam of the argon laser. Burns could be made more effectively with these lasers than with the xenon-arc photocoagulator, but the results of the direct treatment of abnormal vessels were disappointing.

At the same time, an extremely exciting indirect effect of extensive photocoagulation became apparent. This was the regression of new vessels and the resolution of retinal edema and vascular congestion at a distance from the areas being treated. Why these "distant effects" occurred was not understood at the time, and their cause is still not clear. Initially, it was hypothesized that by destroying oxygen-starved cells in the retina, the light also destroyed a vessel-promoting factor. Subsequently, it was proposed that the treatment may destroy the metabolically active portion of the retina containing the photoreceptor cells, thereby allowing better oxygenation of the remaining neural retina. A third possibility is that the pigmented layer of the retina may produce a vessel-inhibiting factor and the "injury" of photocoagulation increases its production.

In spite of these reports of positive indirect effects, by the end of the 1960s there remained considerable disagreement about the effectiveness of xenon-arc or laser photocoagulation. Ederer and Hiller [2] reviewed the early reports concerning photocoagulation and concluded that they suffered from small numbers of patients, brief periods of follow-up, and/or lack of randomly selected control groups.

The National Diabetic Retinopathy Study

By 1971 we had three major questions about the effectiveness of photocoagulation in preserving the vision of patients with proliferative diabetic retinopathy. These were as follows.

1. Does photocoagulation help prevent severe visual loss from proliferative diabetic retinopathy?
2. Is there a difference with respect to efficacy and safety between two treatment techniques: (a) extensive scatter treatment with the *argon laser* plus focal treatment of surface new vessels, elevated new vessels, and new vessels on or near the optic nerve disk, or (b) extensive scatter treatment with the *xenon arc* plus focal treatment of surface new vessels?
3. Are there some stages of retinopathy in which treatment is helpful but others in which it is of no value or harmful?

A problem with earlier studies was that many did not include a comparison of untreated eyes (the *controls*) with treated eyes. In addition, even in the few controlled studies, none followed one of the basic principles of valid clinical trials: the random assignment to treatment or control groups. Finally, a large trial was needed because it was well known that there was considerable variability in the course of proliferative diabetic retinopathy and that dramatic and spontaneous remissions were not uncommon. For these reasons, it was concluded that randomization of a large number of eyes to treatment and control groups was essential to a proper evaluation of photocoagulation as a treatment for this disorder [3, 4].

The National Eye Institute in 1971 funded a study to provide scientifically credible answers to these questions. The timing of this project reflected the level of controversy that existed. Although the technology was present to undertake the trial at an earlier time, it is questionable whether there was sufficient interest and concern on the part of the ophthalmological community to have started one.

Patients included in the study were those with *preretinal* or *intravitreal* new vessels in at least one eye, or with "severe" nonproliferative retinopathy in both eyes, and with visual acuity of 20/100 or better in each eye. These patients were assigned randomly to either the argon or the xenon group. For each patient one eye was selected randomly for prompt photocoagulation treatment. In both groups, treatment consisted in use of the scatter technique, with burns spaced about one-half to one burn width apart extending from the "posterior pole" (the back of the eye where the macula and optic disk are located) to the equator of the globe. Patients received follow-up treatment at four-month intervals as needed. The major endpoint by which the response was judged was *visual acuity.* In addition, the visual field (the area within which the eye can perceive light) and changes in the retina and vitreous gel were also considered in the evaluation of treatment.

The major finding of the Diabetic Retinopathy Study was that *argon-laser and xenon-arc photocoagulation treatment reduce the risk of severe visual loss in patients with moderate to severe diabetic retinopathy* [5]. Severe visual loss was defined by the Diabetic Retinopathy Study as the inability to read the biggest letter on the eye chart at a distance of 5 feet for two consecutive visits. This is equivalent to 5/200 vision, or the ability to read at a distance of 5 feet letters that a normal patient can read at 200 feet. In the Diabetic Retinopathy Study, after two years this degree of visual loss occurred in 6–7 percent of eyes that were treated. In the untreated group, however, vision was reduced to 5/200 in approximately 14 percent of eyes. The difference between severe visual loss in treated and untreated eyes became more dramatic after four years. Severe visual loss was documented in 11 percent of xenon-arc-treated eyes and 13 percent of argon-laser-treated eyes, while between 28 and 30 percent of untreated eyes suffered severe visual loss.

The side effects of photocoagulation treatment were also reported. Described as a loss of ability to read one to four lines of the eye chart, these effects occurred in 9 percent of argon-laser-treated eyes and 20 percent of xenon-arc-treated eyes. In the latter group, approximately 2 percent of eyes experienced this reduction in vision as a result of the treatment. Furthermore, moderate loss of peripheral vision has been attributed to treatment in 40 percent of eyes in this group. Laser treatment was accomplished with minor discomfort and in an office setting.

How do the beneficial and harmful effects balance out? Overall, there was less severe visual loss in the "low-risk" eyes (those with less severe retinopathy), with or without treatment. However, untreated eyes were twice as likely to develop severe visual loss as treated eyes. In the "high-risk" group (those with more severe retinopathy), the benefits of treatment were even more dramatic.

The results of the Diabetic Retinopathy Study led the investigators, and ultimately ophthalmologists in general, to the conclusion that all "high-risk" patients should receive laser photocoagulation treatment [6]. They did so not only because of the strong probability of severe visual loss if these eyes were left untreated, but also because the benefits of treatment clearly outweighed the risks of untoward side effects. Whether prompt photocoagulation treatment or deferral of treatment with careful observation was indicated for eyes with less severe diabetic retinopathy (the "low-risk" category) was not clear.

This study was a monumental undertaking—the largest multicenter trial in the history of eye research. Sixteen major medical centers participated and 1,758 patients were enrolled. Recruitment began in April 1972, and the last patient was enrolled in September 1975. The Diabetic Retinopathy Study received support of a million dollars per year from the National Eye Institute. Its findings, that timely photocoagulation was an effective means of promoting remission and stabilization of diabetic retinopathy, was a dramatic advance in the treatment of a disorder that had often previously progressed relentlessly to blindness.

The Early Treatment of Diabetic Retinopathy Study

The Early Treatment of Diabetic Retinopathy Study (ETDRS) was designed to answer three clinical questions not addressed in the earlier study:

1. When is it most effective to initiate laser photocoagulation treatment in the course of diabetic retinopathy?
2. Can macular edema in diabetes be treated effectively with laser photocoagulation?
3. Does the anticoagulative effect of aspirin alter the course of diabetic retinopathy?

This study [7] demonstrated that early laser photocoagulation was associated with a small reduction in the incidence of visual loss. This effect was quantified in terms of "doubling" of visual acuity (Doubling indicates a loss of vision, as for example when vision goes from 20/20 to 20/40. 20/20 signifies that at a distance of 20 feet an individual can see what a "normal" person sees at 20 feet. 20/40 means that at a distance of 20 feet, the individual sees what a "normal" person would see at 40 feet.) In patients followed for three years without laser treatment, 30 percent experienced a doubling of visual acuity; in contrast, only 15 percent of patients with laser treatment experienced doubling. Because of the adverse effects of photocoagulation, however, laser photocoagulation surgery was not recommended for eyes with mild or moderate non-proliferative diabetic retinopathy.

On the other hand, this study demonstrated that for edema of the critical macular area of the retina, focal laser photocoagulation is effective in reducing the risk of moderate visual loss. Such focal treatment also increases the chance of visual improvement and decreases the frequency of persistent macular edema.

Finally, aspirin treatment did not prevent the development of high-risk proliferative retinopathy or reduce the risk of visual loss; but neither did it increase the risk of vitreous hemorrhage. In other words, aspirin did neither good nor harm.

The Economic Impact of Laser Therapy

In the years from 1972 to 1981, during which the National Eye Institute funded the Diabetic Retinopathy Study, this study cost taxpayers in the United States 10.5 million dollars. When one considers the amount paid by the federal government for blindness-related disability, the savings resulting from the trial are impressive [8]. It is estimated that the trial generated a net saving of 231 million dollars, and when the costs of lost production are added, the net savings increases to 2,816 million dollars for all patients treated with photocoagulation in the 20 years since the onset of the Diabetic Retinopathy Study in 1972. Put in other terms, it gained 279,000 years of vision for the patients who were treated.

In another study of the benefit of eye research using diabetic retinopathy as a model, Javitt and coworkers conclude: "Screening and testing retinopathy in patients with Type I diabetes mellitus was cost effective using all screening strategies. Between 71,000 and 85,000 person-years of sight and between 77,000 and 95,000 person-years of reading vision can be saved for each annual cohort of patients with Type I diabetes mellitus when proper laser photocoagulation is administered. This results in an annual cost savings of $62.1 to 108.6 million" [9]. There is, unfortunately, no additional specific information that we could find at present regarding the effects of treatment on the ability of patients with diabetic retinopathy to work or to carry on basic life functions.

Applying the Lessons of the Diabetic Retinopathy Studies

Much of what we have learned from the diabetic retinopathy treatment studies has not been successfully translated into medical practice. It is clear that new approaches are needed for implementing new policies. Problems exist both with diabetic patients and with physicians. It is not until the condition is advanced that patients suffer decreased vision. Many patients with early diabetic retinopathy do not seek treatment. Delays may occur as a result of denial on the part of the patient; ignorance of the dangers of diabetic retinopathy and/or of the advantages of the treatment available; fears regarding the costs of treatment or of the treatment itself; or lack of access to a center where photocoagulation treatment can be obtained.

Physicians may also stand in the way of early treatment, as when they fail to diagnose diabetic retinopathy: physicians who are not ophthalmologists have been shown to be able to detect proliferative retinopathy under ideal conditions only 50 percent of the time, compared with 90 percent for ophthalmologists and 100 percent for retinal specialists. Detection of diabetic retinopathy is best accomplished by ophthalmoscopic examination by a retina specialist or an experienced ophthalmologist with an interest in diabetic eye disease.

Attempts to counter these problems have led to the analysis of the medical and economic implications of various screening strategies for detecting retinopathy in a diabetic population. The approaches include screening programs carried out at 6-, 12-, and 24-month intervals utilizing various combinations of ophthalmoscopic examination and photography of the fundus of the eye.

Given the savings noted above [8, 9], screening appears to be worthwhile from a societal point of view. Incentives are needed, however, to encourage screening by caregivers such as health maintenance organizations. All of the screening alternatives hold the prospect of saving substantial amounts paid by the federal government for blindness-related disability and preventing loss of productivity due to blindness. The particular frequency and type of screening and the exact population targeted will determine cost-effectiveness. Combining screening with existing care will be a major challenge, and additional study and planning will be needed to make fully available the benefit of laser therapy to the diabetic population.

Editors' Note

This case illustrates the use of a powerful but expensive tool of technology assessment—the multicenter, randomized, controlled clinical trial—to establish whether a treatment is beneficial and whether it may be improved. Because of the irregular, stepwise progression of diabetic retinopathy and the occurrence of partial improvement after treatment, a clinical trial must be rigorously planned and executed if it is to reach a convincing result. It must include concurrent treatment and control groups, preferably assigned randomly; carefully specified treatment protocols; and prolonged follow-up of large numbers of patients. In this context, anecdotal reports of small, uncontrolled series will not provide credible conclusions. Each of these specifications, however, adds to the cost of the trial.

The National Diabetic Retinopathy Study of the efficacy of photocoagulation was the largest clinical trial ever carried out in eye research. At a cost of more than a million dollars per year for ten years, it documented a dramatic advance in the treatment of a condition that was a major cause of blindness. The Early Treatment Study was designed to determine the optimum timing of this treatment. From its results, researchers have defined stages of retinopathy for which there is insufficient net benefit to the patient to justify treatment.

Benefits to the vision of individual patients aside, the taxpayers who support such trials may wish to know what they have received for their money. Although the cost of the first trial was more than ten million dollars, the net savings in program costs for the blind over the ensuing twenty years due to photocoagulation therapy approached a quarter of a billion dollars. The second trial, by demonstrating that some forms of treatment were not efficacious, also saves money over time.

Still, the benefits that can be achieved by photocoagulation treatment of diabetic retinopathy currently are not fully realized. In part this is because retinopathy is not symptomatic during its early and most treatable stages, which means that diabetic patients are unlikely to seek periodic evaluation unless educated to do so. Furthermore, primary caregivers do not accurately recognize diabetic retinopathy, and programs of regular screening by experts, although cost-effective from the societal perspective, are still more likely to be the exception than the rule.

5

The Treatment of Unipolar Depression

Unipolar Depression and the Patient

Most of us are not prepared to recognize or to deal effectively with depression. On the one hand, if we are its victims, the condition itself makes it difficult to seek help. On the other, serious depression in those around us can too easily be interpreted as willful self-deprecation, inactivity, and withdrawal. We, as observers, expect evidence of injury to accompany illness, and we require evidence of energetic self-reliance to disprove malingering. But the individual with severe depression usually is unable to break out of the private world of gloom, anxiety, and feelings of personal worthlessness in order to communicate something of the pain of the illness to bystanders. And we bystanders are not well equipped by our experience to fathom the intensity of the symptoms that go along with the illness.

The obstacles to communication between the depressed and the bystanders make particularly important the descriptions of those few who are gifted in communication and who have passed through the dark landscape of severe depression. One such is William Styron, the distinguished American novelist and playwright, author, among other works, of *Lie Down in Darkness, The Confessions of Nat Turner,* and *Sophie's Choice,* and winner of the Pulitzer Prize, the Prix de Rome, and the Prix Mondial Cino del Duca. In a short memoir appropriately titled *Darkness Visible* [1], Styron helps us see into, and perhaps understand a little better, the grim world of the severely depressed:

> By the time we arrived at the museum, having dealt with heavy traffic,
> it was past four o'clock and my brain had begun to endure its familar

siege: panic and dislocation, and a sense that my thought processes were being engulfed by a toxic and unnameable tide that obliterated any enjoyable response to the living world. This is to say more specifically that instead of pleasure—certainly instead of the pleasure I should be having in this sumptuous showcase of bright genius—I was feeling in my mind a sensation close to, but indescribably different from, actual pain. This leads me to touch again on the elusive nature of such distress. That the word "indescribable" should present itself is not fortuitous, since it has to be emphasized that if the pain were readily describable most of the countless sufferers from this ancient affliction would have been able to confidently depict for their friends and loved ones (even their physicians) some of the actual dimensions of their torment, and perhaps elicit a comprehension that has been generally lacking; such incomprehension has usually been due not to a failure of sympathy but to the basic inability of healthy people to imagine a form of torment so alien to everyday experience. For myself, the pain is most closely connected to drowning or suffocation—but even these images are off the mark. William James, who battled depression for many years, gave up the search for an adequate portrayal, implying its near impossibility when he wrote in *The Varieties of Religious Experience:* "It is a positive and active anguish, a sort of psychical neuralgia wholly unknown to normal life."

Styron's words provide us with an elegant description of the feeling of depression, but for the purposes of this chapter we must also specify the disease in terms physicians use. Here we will be discussing major, endogenous, unipolar depression; this set of qualifiers requires some explanation. *Major* is meant to exclude short, mild episodes of being "down" or "blue." *Endogenous* excludes depression consequent to an external event, such as the loss of a loved one; endogenous depression typically has no identifiable, external cause. *Unipolar* indicates that the mood is consistently depressed, as opposed to alternating with periods of mania in what is labeled "bipolar" or "manic-depressive disorder." Henceforth, in the interests of brevity, *depression* will mean major, endogenous, unipolar depression, unless another meaning is specifically noted.

The standard for the diagnosis of depression is the definition given in the *Diagnostic and Statistical Manual of Mental Disorders, Third Edition*—

Table 5-1. Criteria for diagnosis of major depressive episode.

Diagnosis of a major depressive episode requires that patient experienced five or more of the following attributes during the same two-week period, including either item (1) or (2), from the list below:

1. Depressed mood most every day, most of day
2. Markedly diminished interest and pleasure in all, or almost all, activities
3. Significant weight gain or loss (5% within one month)
4. Insomnia or hypersomnia
5. Psychomotor agitation or retardation
6. Fatigue or loss of energy
7. Feelings of worthlessness or inappropriate guilt
8. Diminished ability to think or concentrate
9. Recurrent thoughts of death
10. Absence of all of the following:
    i. Organic factors
    ii. Bereavement
    iii. Delusions or hallucinations without marked mood symptoms
    iv. Schizophrenia

Source: Adapted with permission from the American Psychiatric Association [6].

Revised, of the American Psychiatric Association (DSM-III-R, 1987). It is summarized in brief form in Table 5-1. We call attention in the text to those reports in which standards for inclusion of subjects differed substantially from these criteria. Our access to the literature on the natural history and treatment of depression was initiated via a list, compiled by Thomas C. Chalmers, of published meta-analyses of randomized clinical trials (RCTs). A meta-analysis is a set of bibliographic and statistical methods for combining the results of independent studies in order to strengthen the conclusions that were drawn from the individual studies. The bibliographies of these articles were then searched for relevant reports in the English language, as was the Medline data base. Priority was given to those studies having explicit criteria for inclusion of subjects, random assignment of subjects to receive the treatment being tested or to the concurrently observed control group of subjects, double blinding, and adequate numbers of subjects in each treatment group. When such studies were not available for each question of interest to us, less rigorous studies were used and appropriate caveats will be noted.

Magnitude of the Problem of Depression

The criteria in Table 5-1 give one a sense of the morbidity associated with an episode of major depression. Individuals who have recovered characterize an episode of depression as an intensely unpleasant experience. As Styron puts it, depression is "gloom crowding in on me, a sense of dread and alienation and, above all, stifling anxiety" [1]. Observers note both the degree of disability the patient has in performing everyday physical activities and social roles, the interaction of depressive symptoms and medical conditions [2], and the risk of suicide [3]. Shortening an episode of depression or reducing the frequency of relapse by medical intervention would certainly be a benefit to the patient.

Estimates of the lifetime risk of depression per 100 people in the United States range from 8.3 to 12.3 for males and 20.3 to 25.8 for females [3], roughly one in ten for men and one in five for women. At any given time in the United States, 3.2 percent of men and 5.2 percent of women are afflicted with depression [4]. Using 1988 data for U.S. population of 121.4 million men and 127.3 million women [5], we estimate the disease burden from depression to be roughly 10.5 million individuals. Approximately half of those who have an initial episode of major depression from which they have recovered will have at least one recurrence [6–8].

What are the risks of depression? Styron tells us that "the pain of severe depression is quite unimaginable to those who have not suffered it, and it kills in many instances because its anguish can no longer be borne. The prevention of many suicides will continue to be hindered until there is a general awareness of the nature of this pain" [1]. In 1988, the overall U.S. annual rate of suicide was 12.3 per 100,000 people [5, 9]. In contrast, among those initially diagnosed as having major depression, the risk of subsequent, successful suicide has been found to be more than fifty times this rate over an average follow-up of six years [10].

In another study, 182 patients hospitalized for depression between 1930 and 1940 were identified, along with a similar, randomly selected control sample of 109 patients admitted concurrently to the same institution for appendectomy and hernia repair. The status of individuals in both groups was determined 30–40 years later. In the group of patients who originally were depressed, 132 had died, 14 by suicide, for an overall suicide rate among the depressed of 10.6 percent. The control population of 109, of whom 37 had died, had no deaths from suicide [11]. Other circumstances being equal, a randomly selected population of 200 people, approximately twice the size of the control group, might be expected to experience one suicide over a forty-year period.

Suicide can be resolution and relief. Styron again:

> At dinner I was barely able to speak, but the quartet of guests, who were all good friends, were aware of my condition and politely ignored my catatonic muteness. Then, after dinner, sitting in the living room, I experienced a curious inner convulsion that I can describe only as despair beyond despair. It came out of the cold night; I did not think such anguish possible.
>
> While my friends quietly chatted in front of the fire I excused myself and went upstairs, where I retrieved my notebook from its special place. Then I went to the kitchen and with gleaming clarity— the clarity of one who knows he is engaged in a solemn rite—I noted all the trademarked legends on the well-advertised articles which I began assembling for the volume's disposal: a new roll of Viva paper towels I opened to wrap up the book, the Scotch-brand tape I encircled it with, the empty Post Raisin Bran box I put the parcel into before taking it outside and stuffing it deep down within the garbage can, which would be emptied the next morning. Fire would have destroyed it faster, but in garbage there was an annihilation of self appropriate, as always, to melancholia's fecund self-humiliation. I felt my heart pounding wildly, like that of a man facing a firing squad, and knew I had made an irreversible decision.   [1]

An approximation of the unmet need for medical care is given by the estimate that more than half of all persons with major depression fail to seek treatment for the episode [12]. Implicit in the use of a phrase like "unmet need," of course, is the assumption that available treatment alters the length or depth of an episode of depression. We turn to this matter next.

The Effect of Treatment on the Initiating Episode of Depression

Descriptions of the natural history of depression or of the effects of treatment must include a time scale with a reference point. In a study that follows a series of patients being treated for depression, some will be suffering from their first episode of depression while others may already have had several episodes of variable length and frequency. We will use the term *initiating episode* for the period of depression that brought the patient to observation and treatment. This episode, which may be the first or the latest of many for that patient, will serve as the reference point for beginning the description of the individual's clinical course.

Given the onset of a major episode of depression, what are the results of the various methods of treatment? Without specific intervention, the episode typically lasts six months or more [6]. In 20 percent or more of initiating episodes, the illness runs a chronic course of continued symptoms whether or not treatment is given [13, 14].

The interventions to be considered here include no treatment (usually achieved by putting the patient on a waiting list for some form of conventional therapy), placebo (an intervention designed to look like the treatment being tested, but which does not have the component of the treatment thought to be active; an example would be a sugar pill made to look exactly like a pill containing the tricyclic antidepressant medication), antidepressant drugs of three types (tricyclics, monoamine oxidase inhibitors, or MAOIs, and lithium), cognitive or behavioral therapy, and electroconvulsive therapy (ECT). Our failure to deal explicitly with some more recent therapies—fluoxetine, for example—should not be interpreted as a vote against these therapies. It means that the information available about the "conventional" treatments is more complete and better illustrates the general points we wish to make.

Most of the studies that are methodologically adequate use remission rates of the initiating episode as the outcome of interest. Typically, a remission means that the patient no longer fulfills the criteria listed in Table 5-1 and, furthermore, has maintained this improvement for a period of eight or more weeks. The probability of relapse after recovery, or the interval to relapse, appears to be influenced by the number of prior episodes of depression [15, 16]. Most series enroll patients whose initiating episode is one in a series of episodes as well as those experiencing depression for the first time, and the inclusion of a variable proportion of subjects who have had prior episodes of depression may confound the observed outcomes.

The meta-analysis by Janicak and coworkers offers the most complete set of comparisons of the major treatments for endogenous depression [17]. They found 22 studies that gave explicit descriptions of the systematic methods for diagnosing depression and determining response to treatment, that used random assignment of subjects to categories of treatment, and that involved single- or double-blind observation—that is, the subject (in a single-blinded trial) or the subject and the person observing the results of treatment (in a double-blinded trial) were unaware whether the subject was receiving treatment or a placebo. For our purposes, the major defect in the meta-analysis is the inclusion of an unspecified number of patients with diagnoses of types of depression other than major, endogenous, unipolar depression.

To test whether the possible heterogeneity of types of depression might alter the treatment outcomes, we compared the results of the meta-analysis with those of a multicentric, controlled, randomized, and blinded trial conducted by the Medical Research Council (MRC) of the United Kingdom. This trial was a study of equivalent interventions and similar endpoints in the treatment of subjects with primary depression [18]. The comparison is presented in Table 5-2. The performance of a pair of treatment modalities is expressed as the difference in the response rates of the two, where the first member of the pair is the intervention with the highest response rate. In the case of the meta-analysis, each expression of efficacy, or net percent of patients improved under research conditions, represents the result of pooling a number of studies of that particular pair of interventions. In the case of the MRC trial, there is only one study with four treatment arms, or three comparisons to placebo. Values for the net efficacy of ECT versus tricyclic antidepressant drugs and ECT versus MAOIs were directly estimated in the meta-analysis. In order to derive estimates of net efficacy for the same pairs of interventions in the MRC study, the appropriate comparisons of treatment to placebo were combined to yield values for the net efficacy of ECT versus tricyclics and ECT versus MAOIs.

Another way of reporting efficacy, not shown in the body of Table 5-2, is to consider the interventions separately, that is, not to compare them to any treatment, including placebo treatment. The meta-analysis of Janicak and colleagues [17] provides the following results expressed as the percent of subjects responding to the treatment: placebo, 45 percent; ECT, 86 percent; tricyclics, 67 percent; and MAOI, 39 percent.

Table 5-2 supports three conclusions. First, the potential heterogeneity of diagnoses in the meta-analysis [17] does not seem to have produced results that are clinically different from those in the MRC study [18]. Second, the net efficacy of ECT over placebo, a response rate of approxi-

Table 5-2. Concurrent comparisons of net efficacy of treatments for depression.

Experimental v. comparison treatments	Net percent improved (number of studies) by source:	
	Janicak et al. [17]	Medical Research Council [18]
ECT[a] v. placebo[d]	41% (5)	32% (1)
ECT v. simulated ECT[d]	32% (6)	Not tested
ECT v. tricyclics[b, d]	20% (7)	19% (1)
ECT v. MAOI[c, d]	45% (5)	41% (1)

a. ECT = Electroconvulsive therapy.

b. Tricyclics = Any member of a chemical family of antidepressant drugs, of which imipramine and amitriptyline are widely used members.

c. MAOI = Monoamine oxidase inhibitors.

d. To underline the meaning of "net efficacy" from a comparison of two modalities, we list here the efficacies of modalities taken one at a time and expressed as percent improved as given in Janicak et al. [17]: placebo, 45%; ECT, 86%; tricyclics, 67%; MAOI, 39%.

mately 40 percent of patients experiencing the initiating episode, is clinically substantial and statistically significant. Third, there is a regular hierarchy of net effect: ECT is better than tricyclics, which are better than MAOI. At a minimum, this regularity is a guide to the most effective therapy. In addition, it informs choice in circumstances where reduced effectiveness must be traded off against reduction in unwanted side effects.

This problem arises in the case of ECT in the following way. Memory loss is the most troubling complication of ECT when treatment is administered to both sides of the brain in the usual fashion. There is widespread agreement that ECT administered only to the nondominant side of the brain (usually the right hemisphere is nondominant in right-handed people) causes less disturbance in memory, but there has been disagreement as to its efficacy in the treatment of major depression. In this connection, an additional meta-analysis reported by Janicak and colleagues is of great interest. Ten published, controlled studies involving 508 subjects were used to compare two-sided ECT to one-sided, nondominant ECT. The average response rates of those treated with two-sided ECT and those treated with one-sided, nondominant ECT were found not to differ significantly [17].

This result is important because it identifies a modification of ECT that is known to have a lower probability of a serious adverse effect than the standard form but is of approximately equal effectiveness. If efficacy of treatment is taken to be the net of benefit and harm, this finding of reduced harm signifies an enhancement in the efficacy of one of the most effective forms of treatment, ECT.

Psychotherapy of a variety of types is another class of interventions that have been used for the treatment of depression. One example, cognitive psychotherapy as developed by Beck and associates [19], is the object of a meta-analysis by Dobson [20]. Once again, a major shortcoming for our purposes is the failure of the analysis to discriminate among the various types of depression of the subjects in the primary reports. In addition, the method of reporting the quantitative performance of the intervention does not permit a direct comparison with the studies quoted earlier. The analysis, however, does support the conclusion that cognitive therapy of depression is superior to no intervention.

A second meta-analysis is directed at comparisons of the effects of five types of psychotherapy and antidepressant drugs [21]. No significant differences in efficacy were found among the categories of psychotherapy. The comparative evaluation of antidepressant drugs was narrowed to one considering all types of psychotherapy versus the most commonly used group of drugs, the tricyclics. Psychotherapy was observed to be superior to tricyclics, but the difference was not statistically significant.

The Effect of Treatment on the Illness-Free Interval

As noted earlier, approximately half of the patients who respond to treatment of an initial episode of depression will have one or more subsequent episodes. Physicians want to know whether what has been called "continuation therapy" affects the probability or timing of relapse. This question raises a number of methodologic issues that are discussed in a helpful review by Belsher and Costello [7].

Two types of evidence can be adduced concerning the pattern of relapse in unipolar depressive disorder. The first brings together information from a number of independent studies on the probability of relapse as a function of time after the initiating episode. The results of twelve such studies noted in the review of Belsher and Costello show that the cumulative probability of relapse increases with time in the first year after recovery from the initiating episode and flattens out thereafter.

The second kind of evidence comes from controlled, randomized clinical trials of continuation therapy after recovery from an initiating episode of depression. Four different interventions were tested in a study by Prien and coworkers: placebo, lithium carbonate, imipramine, and lithium carbonate and imipramine together [22]. For each intervention, the probability of remaining well declined with time, and the risk of relapse per unit of time declined with time after the initiating episode. The results of the two studies thus are consistent.

Of the greatest importance, however, is the clear demonstration that continuation therapy with imipramine, with or without lithium carbonate, improves a patient's prospects for avoiding relapse of depression at least up to 27 months after recovery from the initiating episode. At that time, the probability of remaining well on placebo alone is about 25 percent, whereas the probability is 53 percent on imipramine alone. The effect is clinically substantial and statistically significant. Given the relatively low toxicity of imipramine, the result is strong justification for a period of continuation therapy after the index episode of unipolar depression. An empirically derived, appropriate duration for continuation therapy is not yet established.

Psychotherapy as a form of continuation therapy after a major episode of depression has not been as well studied as have drugs. A single randomized trial of cognitive therapy, medication, or both as initial therapy for the initiating episode and as continuation therapy after recovery showed psychotherapy alone was superior to medication alone [23]. The question merits further study.

Some Financial Consequences of Depression and Its Treatment

One might suspect—from how common depression is, from the recurrence rates even when treatment is provided, and from the possible severity of the symptoms—that the overall costs of treatment and of earnings forgone during periods of illness would be high. We have not been able to find detailed studies of the total financial impact of unipolar depression (as distinct from bipolar depression and dysthymia) in the United States. Our own rough calculations—based on the size of the population, rates of lifetime risk of depression, and the direct and indirect costs of a case from a model developed by Neville and Weinstein [24]—suggest that the annual financial impact of depression in the United States is measured in tens of billions of dollars.

The estimates of the direct and indirect costs of a case of depression by gender and decade of age derived by Neville and Weinstein are of interest from a number of points of view. First, they permit us to put the cost per case in the context of the costs of a number of other common, serious, and aggressively treated diseases. This is illustrated in Figure 5-1, adapted from Neville and Weinstein for the case of a 35-year-old male [24]. The calculations for pulmonary cancer, myocardial infarction or heart attack, and major motor vehicle accident take in the interval from onset to death, while those for depression run from onset to age 65. Despite these methodologic differences, it is apparent that the total costs of care for optimal or best available treatment and typical existing treatment for depression fall well within the range of costs per case for illnesses that we are now treating without questioning the allocation of resources. Although the specific values for costs of treatment and work loss vary somewhat by gender and decade of age, their relative positions among the illnesses chosen for illustration change but little.

A second feature of interest in Figure 5-1 concerns the differences among the direct, indirect, and total costs of treatment for depression in the 35-year-old male. The direct cost of optimal treatment, for example, is several times more than the direct cost of typical treatment, yet total costs, including those due to work loss or forgone income, are, if anything, less than those in the case of typical treatment. We have already noted the medical efficacy of existing treatment for depression. The finding of slightly lower total costs for optimal treatment of depression indicates that, at least for 35-year-old males, optimal treatment not only reduces morbidity but is less expensive from the perspective of total costs. Once again, it is important to remember that total costs, and their partition between treatment and work loss, will vary by gender and decade of life. But the finding in this example of lessened morbidity and lower cost justifies investigation of the cost-effectiveness of treatment across genders and a broader range of ages.

As noted earlier, a substantial fraction, perhaps more than half, of individuals with depression are not treated, perhaps because of the "excruciating near-paralysis" described by Styron [1]. Of those who do come under treatment, not all receive therapy that is considered optimal on the basis of what is known. These two conclusions raise the question of the difference in patient outcome that is achievable by optimal as opposed to typical treatment, and of the difference in total costs between the two approaches to depression.

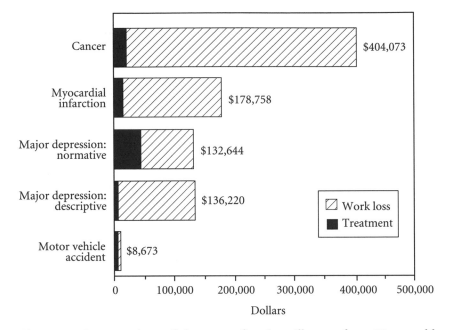

Figure 5-1. A comparison of the costs of various illnesses for a 35-year-old male. Costs are calculated from onset of the condition to death in the cases of pulmonary cancer, myocardial infarction, and major motor vehicle accident, and from onset to age 65 in the cases of major depression treated according to existing practices (descriptive care) and according to consensual standards of optimum care (normative care). Costs are expressed in 1988 dollars, the treatment component of which is standardized using the medical care component of the consumer price index (CPI), and the forgone-earnings component by the general CPI. The costs of depression and the costs of the other examples of illness are not strictly comparable, and the values for work loss and treatment costs will vary somewhat with age and gender. Despite these limitations, the example shows that total costs for an incident case of depression are well within the range of other common illnesses, and that normative treatment of depression, while it changes the partition of costs between treatment and work loss, costs nearly the same as the standard treatment—in this case, less. (Reproduced from an unpublished study by Neville and Weinstein [24] with their permission.)

Table 5-3. Differences in financial costs and health outcomes for an incident case of major depressive disorder receiving typical compared with optimal care.

Gender	Age at start of decade	Additional cost to age 65 due to optimal v. typical care	Additional years without symptoms to age 65 due to optimal v. typical care	Additional cost per additional asymptomatic year
Male	25	($2,402)[a]	1.36[b]	•
	35	($5,107)	1.25	•
	45	($1,722)	1.04	•
	55	($1,980)	0.65	•
Female	25	$12,322	1.40	$8,801
	35	$12,309	1.28	$9,616
	45	$11,944	1.06	$11,268
	55	$9,980	0.68	$14,676

a. The parentheses indicate that the total cost of optimal care minus the total cost of typical care has a negative value, i.e., that optimal care is cheaper than typical care. The figures are in 1987 dollars and are discounted at 5% over the period from onset to age 65.

b. For both genders and for all decades 25 to 65, optimal care increases asymptomatic years as compared with typical care. Years are discounted at 5% over the period from onset to age 65.

Source: Adapted with permission of the author from Tables 6 and 13 in D. Neville [25].

Table 5-3 brings together the relevant results of calculations from a model developed by Neville and Weinstein [25]. For males, the model predicts that optimal treatment results in fewer symptoms *and* lower costs compared with typical treatment. For females, the model predicts significant medical benefits from optimal treatment as well, but at an increase in yearly cost per case over that of typical treatment. The costs per additional asymptomatic year shown in the final column of Table 5-3 are, however, sufficiently low as to argue strongly for optimal treatment of females as well as males.

Policy Concerns

It is clear from recent research that effective treatment exists for depression but that it is underutilized. The analysis sketched in this chapter suggests the merit of two responses from the community at large and the practitioners who are the first line of care. The first response includes heightened awareness of the prevalence of depression, more aggressive case-finding, and more vigorous referral. This response is recommended despite the dilemma sometimes posed by a depressive patient. The dilemma starts with the possibility that the individual not only may fail to seek treatment but may withdraw from offered therapy, leaving the caregiver to decide whether the withdrawal is a life-threatening manifestation of the underlying depression. This dilemma is compounded by the recognition that the individual's withdrawal may be a legitimate exercise of a patient's right to choose among alternative kinds of care, including no care. If the physician is convinced that the patient is a danger to him- or herself, the patient may be compelled to accept treatment, but in this context there is no simple way to balance on behalf of the patient the risks of free choice against the rights of self-determination.

The second response is appreciation of the therapeutic options for depression, and a more sophisticated understanding particularly of the role of treatment with medication. Because many patients will be identified and treated by caregivers other than psychiatrists, the training at least of family practitioners and internists should include additional attention to the recognition of depression and to the availability of effective treatments for it.

Furthermore, since depression is a common condition with high morbidity and high aggregate cost, a strategy directed at prevention is worth seeking. Our understanding of the causes and development of depression is inadequate at present to permit design of a comprehensive program of prevention. Investment in improved understanding, while it does not guarantee future gains in prevention, appears to be a reasonable and highly desirable allocation of research dollars.

Editors' Note

Unipolar depression is a common, chronic, disabling, and potentially fatal disease whose overall burden of illness in our society ranks with that of heart disease. It also is a condition for which there are several kinds of effective treatment. We have confirmed the effectiveness of these treatments because investigators have subjected them to careful clinical trials, as a result of which we can now offer alternative treatments to patients who have adverse reactions to their initial therapy. Our emphasis on controlled trials to evaluate treatments not only makes it possible to draw credible conclusions about the benefits and risks of newer agents, such as fluoxetine, but to realize unappreciated advantages of older treatments, such as unilateral, non-dominant ECT.

Although the demonstration of the efficacy of a treatment is a necessary condition for rational medical care, it is not a sufficient condition. As the case of unipolar depression demonstrates, the potential advantages of effective therapies will be squandered without a realistic and well-supported program of implementation. Such a program will have at least three essential components. First, there must be vigorous and ethically sensitive case-finding, particularly by primary caregivers who recognize the prevalence of depression and who use contemporary screening procedures for its detection. Second, the training of caregivers should include increased emphasis on the proper use of pharmacologic antidepressives in ambulatory care. And third, because unipolar depression is a relapsing illness, the program of care should include some form of continuation therapy and long-term follow-up of the patient.

PART C

Perverse Financial Incentives

In this group of case studies we call attention to two important innovations with great potential for good: kidney transplantation for end stage kidney failure, and the genetically engineered human hormone epoetin for the treatment of certain kinds of severe anemia. For both innovations, the therapeutic potential of the treatments is seriously compromised by perverse incentives built into the reimbursement policies for the two treatments. Reimbursing for only a year's worth of immunosuppressive therapy after kidney transplantation is a dramatic example of a perverse incentive: without immunosuppressive drugs, the patient may reject the transplanted kidney, a waste both of the money spent on the original transplantation and of another scarce resource—the donated organ.

Among the other perverse incentives noted in these chapters is reimbursement for an expensive treatment such as organ transplantation but not for cheaper preventive therapies. This is a problem in the treatment of hypertension, which could prevent some cases of chronic renal failure. Policies concerning employment-related health care insurance may also work against a patient's well-being, as when an individual is able to return to work after treatment for anemia but would risk losing access to continued health care by doing so. Cases such as these highlight the problems we face in the current debate over a national health care policy.

6

Kidney Transplantation

MIRIAM E. ADAMS

Introduction

Chronic kidney failure leading to end stage renal disease (ESRD) is caused by many common diseases, including hypertension and diabetes, and strikes people of all ages. People with ESRD can benefit enormously from medical treatment. The two available treatments—dialysis and kidney transplantation—have successfully saved and currently maintain the lives of nearly 200,000 people in the United States. The potential benefits of the available treatments for ESRD are both enhanced and diminished by societal forces.

In the United States, patients with ESRD can have their medical treatment paid for, up to a point, by the federal Medicare End Stage Renal Disease program. Unfortunately, this program stops funding care just when the treatment has become most effective: one year following transplantation, when the patient is being maintained on immunosuppressive drugs. The number of transplants performed is severely limited by the short supply of donated kidneys, and many potential donations are not realized because of the U.S. policy toward organ donation, culturally based fears, and general lack of knowledge and understanding about organ donation. The result of these forces is an unusual combination in American medical care: an effective treatment for a fatal illness affecting a relatively small number of people, a government program that will cover the cost of treatment regardless of age or economic means of the patient, but a severe limitation on the availability of treatment because of a scarce resource.

End Stage Renal Disease

The two kidneys cleanse the blood of wastes and excess fluids and also perform some endocrine, or hormonal, functions. These organs are essential to life, but humans can survive in good health with only one functioning kidney. When kidney (renal) function deteriorates, as in chronic renal failure, poisonous wastes and potentially toxic substances accumulate in the blood and other body fluids. Patients with renal failure may experience weakness, confusion, nausea, vomiting, fever, and signs and symptoms of toxic effects in almost every organ system. In almost all cases, chronic renal failure eventually reaches the fatal condition of end stage renal disease (ESRD) [1, 2].

In the United States, at least 40,500 people were newly treated for ESRD in 1989. The federal Medicare program that pays for ESRD treatment estimates that the annual number of new patients will increase to nearly 57,000 in the year 2000. In that year, there may be a total of nearly 250,000 patients receiving treatment for ESRD through the Medicare program [3].

Patients who develop ESRD will die if not treated. Modern medicine offers two forms of treatment that take over (though imperfectly) for the nonfunctioning kidneys: hemodialysis and kidney transplantation. Patients generally receive dialysis as the first treatment, with transplantation performed when possible.

Dialysis

The process of dialysis, filtering and cleansing the patient's blood, is most commonly done by machine. Blood flows through a tube from the patient into the dialysis machine, where it is filtered of wastes and toxins, and then the cleansed blood flows back into the patient's arm via another tube. Patients typically spend three to six hours hooked up to the machine during three dialysis sessions each week. In the United States, although some patients have dialysis machines at home or may be treated in hospitals when acutely ill, most go to dialysis centers for their treatments.

For an alternative form of dialysis, peritoneal dialysis, the patient wears an indwelling tube so that fluid can be cycled in and out of the abdominal cavity, where it picks up wastes from the body fluids. Peritoneal dialysis can be performed by machine during several sessions per week. A related option is chronic ambulatory peritoneal dialysis: the patient connects a plastic bag of fluid to the tube, allows the fluid to run slowly into the abdomen, and then uses the empty bag to collect the fluid as it drains back out through the tube. This technique, requiring four 30-minute sessions per day, provides a slow, continuous dialysis.

Conventional dialysis by machine can be a grueling process. It has been said to transform ESRD from a terminal to an interminable illness [2]. Patients must carefully restrict their dietary and fluid intake. The changes in body-fluid composition and rapid removal of salt and fluid from the body during machine dialysis may cause nausea, vomiting, muscle cramps, headache, and sudden drops in blood pressure.

Although dialysis removes many toxic substances from the blood, some toxins, especially those of large molecular weight, remain in the blood after dialysis treatment. This probably accounts for the symptoms and effects of ESRD that may persist in patients receiving dialysis, such as pericarditis (inflammation of the lining around the heart) and neuropathy (abnormal functioning of the peripheral nerves). Dialysis also does not replace other kidney functions, such as the production of the hormone erythropoietin (essential to the bone marrow's production of red blood cells), and production of the active form of vitamin D. Because of these deficits, patients undergoing dialysis treatment may continue to suffer from anemia and bone disease (we refer the reader to Chapter 7 for more information on erythropoietin in ESRD).

A variety of other problems may plague the dialysis patient. Cumulative blood loss caused by machine dialysis (several milliliters per session) can contribute to anemia in dialysis patients. Dialysis may aggravate diabetic disease of the retina (see Chapter 4 for more information on diabetic retinopathy). It may pose some risk to patients with cardiovascular insufficiency, because of the potential for the blood pressure to fall during dialysis treatment. Rapid and severe drops in blood pressure may compromise blood flow through diseased coronary arteries, leading to myocardial infarction (heart attack). Dialysis patients are often sterile, and men may develop impotence. Children receiving dialysis may have problems with growth and development.

Chronic ambulatory peritoneal dialysis is much less grueling than conventional machine dialysis, permits a normal diet, and does not result in the blood loss common in machine dialysis. Chronic ambulatory peritoneal dialysis has a survival rate comparable to that of machine dialysis performed in hospitals or dialysis centers. Because it is slower and more nearly continuous than machine dialysis, it helps to maintain steady-state body-fluid levels. The main risk associated with the treatment is peritonitis, bacterial infection of the peritoneum. Patients undergoing chronic ambulatory peritoneal dialysis average one to two such infections per year [1].

Dialysis does not cure kidney disease and does not return patients with end stage renal disease to a state of robust good health. It does, however, rescue patients with kidney failure from certain death, enabling many of them to continue with the usual activities of daily life.

Kidney Transplantation

The first successful kidney transplant in humans was done in 1954 in Boston. The recipient, the identical twin of the donor, survived for nine years with normal kidney function before dying of a heart attack [4]. Transplants between identical twins are ideal (and most likely to be successful) because the transplanted organ will not be rejected by the host. Unfortunately, most kidney patients in need of a transplant must rely on other sources of donation. Kidneys may be transplanted from any donor whose genetic make-up closely matches that of the recipient. Donors may be family members, or unrelated to the recipient, and they may be living or dead (cadaveric donors). Organs donated by other than an identical twin will be rejected by the recipient's immune system unless the immunologic response is inhibited, usually by immunosuppressive drugs. The greatest obstacle to successful kidney transplantation is the immunological barrier; the technical aspects of kidney transplantation surgery have been resolved.

In kidney transplantation surgery, the kidney is excised from the donor, along with its artery, vein, and ureter, and placed in the recipient's pelvis. The artery and vein are joined to large blood vessels, and the ureter is joined to the recipient's bladder. The transplanted kidney is well protected by the surrounding bones and abdominal muscles in the pelvic area.

Developments in surgical techniques and immunosuppression have improved safety and efficacy of kidney transplantation, making transplantation the treatment of choice for ESRD. As transplantation has become more successful, the selection criteria for possible recipients have been relaxed, so that the majority of patients with ESRD are now considered suitable for transplantation. The clinical barriers to performing transplants in older or diabetic patients have diminished over the past decade. A diabetic transplant patient now does better than a diabetic dialysis patient, but not as well as a nondiabetic transplant patient. Generally, dialysis patients in the United States will be placed on the waiting list for transplantation unless transplantation is medically futile or the patient wishes to continue with dialysis.

The ethics of providing transplantation to elderly patients are still debated, and in 1989, only 2 percent of kidney transplant recipients in the United States were 65 years of age or older.

Immunosuppressive Treatment after Transplantation

As noted earlier, the leading cause of loss of a transplanted kidney is rejection by the recipient's body. Rejection is a complex immunologic response to incompatible donor-tissue proteins that occurs when donor and recipient are imperfectly matched. The clinical manifestations of rejection range from an asymptomatic reduction in kidney function to acute kidney failure, hypertension, and coagulation of blood throughout the body. In addition to loss of the transplanted kidney, rejection can sometimes lead to the death of the recipient. To prevent rejection, transplant recipients must take drugs that suppress immune function for the rest of their lives.

Cyclosporine A became established during the 1980s as the foundation of immunosuppressive therapy. It produces better long-term survival of transplanted organs than the alternative treatment of azathioprine and steroids. Cyclosporine does not indiscriminately reduce the immune system's defenses against infection; rather, it reduces immune defenses only against foreign tissue. Cyclosporine's major drawback is that it is toxic to the kidneys, and this effect may be difficult to distinguish from rejection of the transplanted organ.

Cyclosporine is also expensive, and the cost must be borne over the patient's remaining lifetime. This is the one aspect of ESRD treatment that the Medicare ESRD program does not cover; one year after a successful transplantation, the patient must begin paying for the immunosuppressive drugs. For some patients, this may be an overwhelming financial burden, and may compromise the effectiveness of their treatment. New agents are being developed, but most of those in widest use are expensive. This gap in coverage of kidney-transplant patients illustrates how a detail of reimbursement policy may be at odds with the overall thrust of the parent policy. The result is potential waste of a scarce resource, the donated kidneys, and unnecessary risk and discomfort for the patient.

Case Vignette: Affording Immunosuppression

Albert Isaac is a 36-year-old computer programmer who, with his wife, is guardian and parent to eight foster children. Three years ago, Mr. Isaac started dialysis treatment for end stage renal failure. After a year on dialysis, he received a kidney donated by a brother. Despite the fact that the transplant met only the minimum standards for immunologic compatibility, he showed no signs of transplant rejection. His program of immunosuppressive medication included the most effective available agent, cyclosporine, whose $7,000 annual cost was covered by the federal ESRD program for the first year.

The ESRD entitlement for immunosuppressive drugs expires one year after transplantation, even though failure to continue immunosuppression usually will cause rejection and loss of the transplanted kidney, whose costs originally were paid for by the ESRD program. During the second post-transplant year, Mr. Isaac's cyclosporine costs were covered by his work-related health insurance, but then he was notified that his employer was changing insurers and that the new one would not continue the medication coverage in the third post-transplant year.

Knowing that he could not manage the annual cost of the cyclosporine as an out-of-pocket expense, Mr. Isaac took two actions. First, using his second-year coverage, he built up a modest stockpile of the cyclosporine. Second, he asked his physician to develop a schedule for the gradual substitution of other, albeit less effective, immunosuppressive drugs for the cyclosporine during the third year following the transplant, the plan being to terminate use of cyclosporine thereafter. This schedule is now being implemented.

The restrictions surrounding coverage of immunosuppressive drugs more than a year after transplantation put at risk of rejection his currently functioning kidney. It also, perversely, threatens the investment already made in procuring the donor kidney and transplanting it into Mr. Isaacs.

Quality of Life and Health Following Transplantation

Transplantation, when successful, restores a patient to a more satisfactory quality of life than dialysis does, with greater physical and mental vigor and freedom from the rigors of the dialysis routine. Yet, the quality of life for transplant patients is not ideal, for they must always live with the uncertainty that their transplanted kidney may fail at any time. Transplant recipients often must take a plethora of medications, including antibiotics, anticonvulsive agents, antihypertensives, and diuretics, in addition to the immunosuppresive agents mentioned earlier. Studies of transplant recipients have shown that 75–80 percent of recipients with functioning grafts live virtually normal lives, but the same could be said of only 25–60 percent of dialysis patients [4].

Kidney transplant recipients are likely to experience depression and anxiety, especially in response to complications. Psychiatric illness, including major depression and psychosis, occurs in up to 32 percent of recipients, and there is a higher suicide rate among transplant recipients than among the general population.

Long-term studies of patients with functioning transplanted kidneys over five years show that 94 percent suffer from some late complications, such as hypertension and cataracts [4]. Because of the immunosuppressive therapy, transplant recipients have a very high incidence of certain cancers, such as cancer of the skin, lips, vulva, and anus, non-Hodgkin's lymphoma, and Kaposi's sarcoma. Annual mortality among kidney transplant recipients is from 4 to 7 percent.

Case Vignette: ESRD and Diabetes

Because kidney failure often results from chronic diseases such as hypertension and diabetes, ESRD patients tend to have complex medical problems that complicate the treatment decision and that may affect the patient's potential for rehabilitation after transplantation. Still, kidney transplantation can be highly effective for such complicated cases, and, as in the case of Marie Ritelli, the underlying diabetes can sometimes be treated simultaneously. (Like the subjects of all the case vignettes presented in this chapter, Marie Ritelli is a fictitious, but typical, ESRD patient.)

Marie Ritelli is a 31-year-old single woman who is the office manager for a small firm that provides financial counseling and estate-planning services to individual investors. She has had diabetes, requiring insulin treatments since early childhood, but she finished school and worked steadily until just after her thirty-first birthday, when she began to be troubled by chronic fatigue, loss of appetite and weight, and episodes of nausea and vomiting. Medical evaluation shows the cause of her symptoms to be severe kidney failure due to diabetes. She was immediately put on dialysis as a lifesaving measure while she and her physicians explore the options for her subsequent treatment.

Further examination showed irreversible blindness in one eye from diabetic changes in the small blood vessels, and moderate changes in the blood vessels of the other eye (we refer the reader to Chapter 4 for more information on diabetic retinopathy). Although she is able to read printed material with her good eye, her vision is not good enough so that she feels able to drive. She has no cardiac symptoms, but an exercise test shows that part of her heart muscle may not be receiving adequate amounts of blood, increasing her risk of a heart attack. Neurologic testing shows a decrease in feeling in her lower legs and feet, another complication of her long-standing diabetes. Given the likelihood of further complications due to diabetes, the choice of treatment for her kidney failure is between the inconvenient but relatively less traumatic option of dialysis and the commitment of a scarce resource—a donated organ—to the major and complex treatment by transplantation.

Ms. Ritelli accepted the recommendation that she have a combined kidney and pancreas transplant with the hope that it would treat both her kidney failure and her diabetes. Her postoperative course was complicated by two episodes of immune damage to her transplants and an episode of depression requiring hospitalization, but fifteen weeks after her surgery she returned full-time to her old job.

Other Barriers to Successful Transplantation

In 1989, nearly 9,000 kidney transplantations were performed in the United States. Approximately 20 percent of these kidneys were from living related donors, 78 percent were from cadaveric donors, and the remaining came from living donors unrelated to the recipients [3]. The annual number of kidney transplants increased steadily from the early 1970s through 1986, then leveled off through 1990. This is probably due to the very limited supply of organs. In fact, the supply of donated kidneys poses the greatest barrier to patients seeking kidney transplants. Other factors—such as quality of the match, socioeconomic factors, and patient compliance with the treatment regimen—contribute to the success of the procedure.

At some transplant centers, the median waiting time for a kidney transplant is as long as 71 months for first transplants, although on average in the United States patients wait less than a year to receive a kidney [3]. Waiting times for people of color and for women tend to be longer, because it is more difficult to find compatible kidneys for these groups given the limitations of the existing supply. Women who have been pregnant become more highly sensitized to a wide range of antigens. Racial differences in blood groups and other genetic factors make it more likely that a well-matched kidney will come from a member of the same race. A relative lack of minority organ donors severely limits the number of well-matched kidneys available for minority recipients [5].

African Americans with ESRD are faced with fewer opportunities for transplantation and poorer kidney-survival rates after transplantation than White Americans. In terms of the risk of developing ESRD, the incidence of ESRD in Blacks is four times greater than in Whites. Adult Native Americans also have a higher risk of ESRD: three times higher than for Whites. Higher risk may also exist among Latinos, but studies have found conflicting results. These racial differences in incidence of ESRD have not been fully explained but are related to the significantly higher incidence of hypertension leading to kidney damage among Blacks (52 percent of Black Americans with hypertension develop kidney damage, compared with 8 percent of White hypertensives) [6]. The higher rates may also be related to socioeconomic factors [3, 5].

Thirty percent of patients on waiting lists for donated kidneys are Black, and they must wait nearly twice as long as White patients to obtain a kidney. While Blacks receive over 22 percent of the kidneys available from cadaveric donors, they make up only about 8 percent of cadaveric donors [3]. Some of the common reasons that Black Americans choose not to donate organs include lack of awareness about transplantation, religious beliefs, distrust of the medical community, and fear of premature death [7].

Following transplantation, Black recipients have survival rates of the transplanted kidney that are 10–20 percent lower than for any other ethnic group. Two years after receiving kidneys from living, related donors, the kidney-survival rate is 75 percent for Blacks and 89 percent for Whites [7]. This difference reflects losses due to the recipients' inability to obtain information or to afford medications, as well as other sociologic effects. Despite the difference in kidney survival after transplantation, there are no reported differences in patient survival between Black and White Americans.

Maximizing the Benefits of Kidney Transplantation

How many ESRD patients could potentially benefit from a kidney transplant? One estimate, using 1988 data, gave a range of 11,000 to 16,000 patients who might be suitable for transplantation, of the 22,300 new

ESRD patients under age 65 in that year [3]. This is substantially more than the approximately 8,800 kidney transplants done in that year. By the end of 1989, over 16,000 names were on waiting lists for kidney transplants [3]. The number of donated organs falls far short of the potential number of recipients. Only about 35 percent of all potential cadaveric donors actually provide organs.

Increasing the number of organ donors, especially among minorities, would increase the number of patients able to receive transplantation. A larger, more diverse pool of donated organs would also enhance survival of transplanted kidneys, because of improved matching. The donor pool could be increased through increased public and professional education, improved processes for requesting donation from families of potential donors, encouragement of living donation from both related and nonrelated sources, and, eventually, changes in U.S. public policy as described next.

Policymakers might increase the supply of donated kidneys by adopting a policy of presumed consent. This policy, followed in several European countries, vests the government with authority to take cadaveric organs unless the individual has explicitly expressed wishes to the contrary [3]. Presumed consent has been enacted in several areas of the United States only for pituitary glands and corneas. Its enactment for kidneys would go a long way toward meeting the needs of the 11,000 to 16,000 new ESRD patients who are potentially suitable candidates for transplantation each year. As yet, however, presumed consent for kidney donation has not garnered sufficient public support to achieve enactment into law. Given the American dislike for government involvement in such matters, it seems unlikely that presumed consent will be enacted in the near future. Unfortunately, the current policy, requiring hospitals to identify and refer all potential organ donors, does not seem to be very effective, perhaps because of the psychological and sociological barriers to donation.

The pool of donated kidneys could also be enhanced by increasing the number of living donors. The risk to live donors is about equal to the risk of death from commuting 16 miles a day by car. There is no obvious decrease in long-term survival of live donors, once past the period of short-term risk related to surgery. In addition, there probably is no increased incidence of hypertension or renal failure in kidney donors. Serious treatable complications occur in 2–3 percent of donors [4, 8]. Approximately twenty donor deaths have occurred, however, and some opponents of attempts to encourage live donation argue that even one death is too many among healthy donors. Opponents also fear that potential donors could be coerced to consent to donate. Whether for coercion or incentive, it is illegal for money to be involved in organ donation; the National Organ Transplant Act of 1984 made the buying and selling of organs a felony, punishable by a fine of up to $50,000 and a prison term of up to five years. Without some form of incentives, it seems unlikely that the number of unrelated living donors will increase substantially.

Health Policy Issues

Treating end stage renal disease presents many challenging health policy questions about paying for care and determining who should receive these benefits. These questions will become increasingly troubling as the medical technology becomes even more complex.

A major question relates to the allocation of federal funds for treatment versus prevention of disease. The federal government currently pays for all treatment of end stage renal disease but does not similarly cover preventive medical care that could reduce the occurrence or the severity of kidney disease. If all Americans received care for hypertension and diabetes, before complications developed, fewer people would require costly treatment for ESRD. Without universal health care coverage, it is unlikely that an effective prevention program can be implemented in the United States, because so many people have no health insurance and cannot afford routine health care.

Lessons from other countries will teach us something about what is possible, and about what compromises must be made. In the United Kingdom, for example, basic health care is available to all, but more costly technologies, such as treatment for end stage renal disease, are rationed on the basis of age and other complicating conditions. Since the late 1970s, the dominant treatment in the U.K. has been transplantation, while hospital or center dialysis is reserved for patients who have temporary difficulty with home dialysis or with chronic ambulatory peritoneal dialysis and for a small number of others. The U.K. is a leader in kidney transplantation, chronic ambulatory peritoneal dialysis, and home dialysis, while utilization of hospital/center dialysis purposely is kept low. In the United States, such rationing may be thought desirable in the future, but it probably will be very difficult to institute.

In the meanwhile, the demand for kidney transplantation will continue to outstrip the supply of donated kidneys, especially in the United States and in other countries where there is no policy of presumed consent. The benefits of transplantation over dialysis will continue to grow as safer and more effective immunosuppressive therapies are developed. By the twenty-first century, the efforts now under way to develop alternatives to the human kidney for transplantation may prove successful. For example, successful xenografts (kidneys transplanted from animals) or implantation of small bionic dialyzers might become commonplace treatments for ESRD.

As new approaches to ESRD treatment are developed, society will be faced with questions about who will pay and, perhaps, who will directly benefit. By 1990, annual expenditures on the ESRD program in the United States were well over $3 billion. With new, expensive technologies on the horizon, these expenditures are unlikely to decrease. Undoubtedly, as effective artificial alternatives to human kidneys become available, the benefits of ESRD treatment will be limited less by the paucity of organ donors than by the scarcity of economic resources.

Editors' Note

The description in 1901 of the now-familiar ABO blood groups made possible the simplest kind of transplantation: blood transfusion. The clinical use of transplantation of solid organs began in 1954, with the successful transplantation of a kidney, as noted in this chapter, from a healthy male to his identical twin with end stage renal disease. Several circumstances contributed to the subsequent effort to extend this dramatic accomplishment to donors and recipients who were unrelated. First, a modicum of kidney function (or its therapeutic equivalent) is essential to continued life; second, the kidney is a paired organ, one of which is more than adequate to sustain normal life; third, the surgical technology of removal and implantation of a kidney is straightforward; fourth, treatment by dialysis permits metabolic preparation of the patient with ESRD for transplantation and can tide the patient over periods of poor function in the donated kidney after transplanation; and fifth, although our understanding of and control over the immunological rejection of transplanted tissue is severely limited, our knowledge base is improving and succeeding generations of immunosuppressive drugs are more selective.

Since its inception in 1973, the U.S. ESRD program has added hundreds of thousands of life-years to the population of patients with chronic kidney failure, largely as the result of continued trials of modifications of immunosuppression therapy. Experience with this condition has exposed some of the difficulties in planning and implementing large-scale service programs. Some of these problems are brought out in this chapter. First, what had been a serious shortage of funds for lifesaving services before the ESRD program was established became a serious shortage of another kind (donor kidneys for transplantation) afterward. Second, long-range estimates of the size of the ESRD program, hence its funding requirements, proved inaccurate because of a progressive broadening of the selection criteria for candidates for treatment. Third, in an effort to better control the costs of the program, reimbursement regulations were established that limited coverage for essential drugs to one year after transplantation. These regulations created perverse financial incentives and compromised care for some patients: for want of a secure supply of drugs, a kidney might be lost and the very expensive cycle of treatment—dialysis, a new transplant—might begin anew.

Kidney transplantation is simply one of what will be a varied portfolio of organ transplants. As an early example, it has much to teach us. First, the creation of an organ-specific program of medical services compartmentalizes health care in an inefficient way. Patients, for example, are entitled to treatment of ESRD brought on by uncontrolled hypertension, but not for the cheaper and superior antihypertensive treatment that could have prevented the development of ESRD in the first place. Second, the incentives built into the program of care must be constructed so that they do not frustrate the fundamental purpose of the program. Severe limitations on the duration of support for immunosuppressive drugs after kidney transplantation is an example of a reimbursement policy at odds with its parent program. Third, the paucity of donated kidneys is now the major constraint on transplantation. As a consequence, optimum therapy cannot be offered to many individuals with ESRD. In addition, the chance for a good immunological match between donor and recipient is enhanced when the pool of donor organs is increased. Low rates of organ donation, particularly in some ethnic groups, cause longer waits for suitable matches for ESRD patients in those groups. Policies such as presumed consent for organ donation would increase the yield of suitable kidneys.

7

Epoetin Therapy for Renal Anemia: Health Policy and Quality-of-Life Perspectives

JENNIFER F. TAYLOR

Introduction

Coping with chronic kidney failure involves more than adjusting to a regimen of thrice-weekly dialysis treatments, dietary restrictions, and long-term medications. J.D. (a fictional character representing the composite experience of many patients with end stage renal disease, or ESRD, treated with epoetin) is a diabetic woman in her early fifties. She is one of the approximately 200,000 patients in the United States whose kidney damage has progressed to the "end stage." The failure of her kidneys has created another problem. They no longer produce enough of a hormone, erythropoietin, which stimulates production of red blood cells by the bone marrow. As a result, the patient becomes anemic, a condition characterized by inadequate oxygen delivery to the body due to an insufficient number of red blood cells. Individuals with anemia often report feeling cold, tired, lethargic, and less alert than normal.

In J.D.'s case, renal anemia had forced her to reduce her daily activities because of her physical weakness and fatigue. Although she had been able to work for more than four years after her kidney failure was initially diagnosed, J.D. eventually had to give up her job, and with it her employer-based health insurance plan. She now depends on Social Security disability payments for income and Medicare for coverage of her medical expenses under a special entitlement program that serves all ESRD patients who are eligible for Social Security benefits, regardless of age.

Because J.D.'s anemia and renal failure caused fatigue, irritability, and mental confusion, her social activities dwindled and many of her friendships dissolved. Her family had tried to minimize her limitations by taking on additional duties, including shopping and housework, but their attempts increased her depression and sense of helplessness.

Initially, J.D.'s nephrologist treated her anemia with steroid medications, but the side effects of the medications (including weight gain, muscle soreness, acne, and the growth of facial hair), made her more self-conscious, while the drugs themselves were only minimally effective.

After the steroids were discontinued, she relied on blood transfusions to correct her anemia. Her need for these transfusions had increased over time so that, on average, she required one transfusion every six weeks. This caused her to worry about the risk of contracting hepatitis or the AIDS virus from the transfused blood, despite her doctor's assurances that blood supplies were rigorously tested. At times she considered abandoning dialysis completely. That decision would have rapidly led to her death from uremic poisoning.

In November 1989, on the advice of her nephrologist, J.D. began taking epoetin, an artificial analog of the hormone erythropoietin normally produced by the kidney. As her nephrologist explained, this drug reversed anemia associated with ESRD in approximately 95 percent of patients, reduced or eliminated their dependence on blood transfusions, and enhanced their quality of life.

Quality of life refers to the ability of individuals to care for themselves, work, enjoy their leisure time, and participate in social and family activities. Patients treated with epoetin report improvements in all these areas, along with improved energy and activity levels, better sleep and sexual functioning, and an increased sense of well-being.

Within nine weeks of beginning the drug program, J.D. began to feel revitalized. Her family noticed that she was more cheerful and optimistic. She and her husband said that after nearly a year's total abstinence, they had resumed sexual activity. In addition, she was seeing friends once again.

Unfortunately, epoetin is very expensive. In J.D.'s case, epoetin therapy costs roughly $6,000 per year. The Medicare ESRD program pays 80 percent of this cost; she is responsible for the remaining 20 percent, or nearly $1,200 per year.

The development of epoetin has revolutionized the treatment of patients with ESRD. It has placed new demands on dialysis centers to schedule treatments during more evening and weekend hours, for patients who have returned to work or who are more active during the day, and to provide more patient education in the area of self-care. It has also allowed patients to take greater control of their lives and the treatment of their renal failure.

This chapter examines the impact of epoetin on the clinical status and quality of life of patients with renal anemia. It also examines the impact of different epoetin reimbursement guidelines set forth by the Health Care Financing Administration (HCFA), the federal agency responsible for regulating the Medicare ESRD program, and some of the barriers that may prevent epoetin-treated patients from realizing their full potential.

End Stage Renal Disease and Renal Anemia

ESRD is caused by a variety of diseases, such as diabetes, hypertension, or kidney stones. Patients with ESRD develop the symptoms noted earlier, due either to the retention of uremic toxins or to anemia, and must rely on a kidney transplant or some form of dialysis to remove uremic toxins from the body; without treatment they would die from the lethal buildup of these waste products.

Most ESRD patients hope for a kidney transplant. Transplant recipients generally function at nearly normal levels, and their quality of life is higher than that of dialysis patients (see Chapter 6). However, only 25 percent of ESRD patients will ever receive a transplanted kidney [1], primarily because of the limited number of available and immunologically compatible donor kidneys. The rest will require some form of dialysis.

Although dialysis prevents a lethal buildup of uremic toxins, it does not reverse the anemia associated with chronic renal failure. Approximately 97 percent of dialysis patients suffer from some degree of anemia. At least 25 percent of these patients have anemia severe enough to require periodic blood transfusions [2], in some patients as often as every four to six weeks. Anemia is probably the foremost reason why only one-third of chronic renal failure patients on dialysis are able to resume their daily activities [2]. The symptoms of anemia are due to an insufficient number of red blood cells carrying oxygen throughout the body. Other factors that may contribute to the severity of anemia in ESRD patients include the presence of uremic toxins, shortened survival times for red blood cells, iron deficiency, and excess aluminum, derived from certain medications, that block bone marrow response to erythropoietin.

Clinical Benefits and Adverse Effects of Epoetin

Epoetin, also called recombinant human erythropoietin, is a genetically engineered version of the naturally occurring human hormone, erythropoietin. Epoetin does not restore the filtering function of the kidneys or reduce patients' dialysis requirements. Clinical trials have shown that epoetin ameliorates renal anemia within eight to twelve weeks, raising the hematocrit (the ratio of the volume of red blood cells to the total volume of blood in a sample) to 30–35 percent in approximately 95 percent of patients [3]. This typically reduces symptoms of anemia, including fatigue, coldness, poor appetite, insomnia, and depression. Bringing the hematocrit closer to the normal range, 37–45 percent, also eliminates or reduces the need for blood transfusions and the small risk of exposure to serious viral diseases.

In a U.S. multicenter study of renal anemia in 247 patients, 51 percent were transfusion-dependent prior to epoetin therapy and required an average of one unit of blood per month. After four months of epoetin therapy, only 1 percent of patients continued to require transfusions [4].

In another U.S. multicenter study of 333 patients treated with epoetin, Eschbach and his colleagues found that of the 174 patients who required almost one transfusion per month during the six-month period prior to treatment, none required blood transfusions after two months of epoetin therapy because their anemia had been corrected by epoetin [3].

Epoetin has its own problems, however. There is increased risk of developing hypertension, or of its exacerbation, in epoetin-treated patients [5]. Although these elevations have been associated with seizures (sudden neurologic dysfunctions caused by abnormalities in the electrical activity of the brain), in clinical studies the annual incidence of seizures among epoetin-treated patients is no greater than that of the general dialysis population (8 percent) [6].

Another potential side effect of epoetin is increased blood clotting at the blood access site for hemodialysis or in other blood vessels, which may lead to heart attack or stroke. Some researchers have found that clotting at the access site occurred in approximately 2 percent of placebo-treated patients and 7 percent of epoetin-treated patients [7].

Quality-of-Life Benefits of Epoetin Therapy

Using a variety of measures and strategies, researchers have charted the impact of medical treatment on patients' everyday lives. Some measures relate to the specific experience of patients with ESRD; others assess more global aspects of well-being. Many studies have combined both types of measures with clinical information for a fuller assessment of the impact of epoetin therapy.

In a placebo-controlled Canadian multicenter study [8] of the impact of epoetin therapy on 118 dialysis patients, investigators used the Kidney Disease Questionnaire, the Sickness Impact Profile (SIP), the time trade-off technique, and objective measures of patients' functional abilities, such as exercise testing.

The Kidney Disease Questionnaire was used to assess the effect of epoetin on specific problems identified by renal patients. It asks questions in five main areas: physical symptoms, fatigue, depression, relationships, and frustration. Patients respond to multiple-choice questions, such as "In the past two weeks, how much energy have you had?" on a scale yielding one point for "no energy at all" to seven points for "full of energy." When the average score on such a question increases by even one-half point in a treated group of sufficient size, the gain is regarded as small but clinically important.

The SIP [9] is a general measure of health status that is used to evaluate health-related dysfunction in twelve areas: social relationships, emotional behavior, alertness behavior, body care and movement, home management, mobility, ambulation, sleep and rest, eating, communication, work, and recreation and pastimes. The SIP yields an overall score of functional ability as well as scores on physical and psychosocial dimensions, which are converted to percentages. Higher percentages indicate greater levels of dysfunction. Global SIP scores for general populations of primarily well adults are approximately 3 percent, indicating low levels of dysfunction [10]. Changes in SIP scores of at least 3–5 percent are clinically important.

In the Canadian study, after six months of therapy, patients in the high-dose epoetin group experienced clinically important positive changes in the areas of physical symptoms, fatigue, depression, and interpersonal relationships, as indicated by responses to the Kidney Disease Questionnaire [8].

Global SIP scores for patients in the study changed from 12.2 percent to 4.4 percent, reflecting a clinically important improvement in patients' overall functional ability. Physical-dimension scores at the six-month follow-up also revealed substantial improvements and were within the normal range for primarily well adults [8].

At the end of the six-month randomized phase of the study, researchers offered all study participants epoetin therapy and extended the follow-up period to eighteen months. Improvements in quality of life were maintained by patients originally assigned to the epoetin groups. Placebo patients who were switched to epoetin therapy also demonstrated subsequent improvements in their quality of life.

A U.S. multicenter study by Evans and his associates [11] found that after ten months of epoetin therapy, only 22 percent of patients complained of having "low" or "no energy," compared with 46 percent before therapy began. This study also used the Nottingham Health Profile to evaluate functioning in the dimensions of pain, emotional reactions, sleep, social isolation, and physical mobility, as well as task performance in areas most affected by health. These include occupational demands, the ability to perform tasks around the home, personal relationships, sexual activity, social activities, hobbies, and leisure activities. A score of 0 indicates no limitations; a score of 100 indicates complete limitation. A decrease in score represents an improvement in clinical status. Average Nottingham Health Profile scores were 50.4 pre-therapy and 23.4 post-therapy. Epoetin-treated patients also reported increased energy and increased ability to perform tasks around the house, to engage in sexual activities, and to engage in hobbies.

These findings reflect decreases in the levels of impairment and improvement in quality of life across a wide range of dimensions reported by patients treated with epoetin. Examining specific areas of quality of life assessed by several studies gives us a more nearly complete picture of the effects of epoetin therapy within specific dimensions.

Patients with ESRD often report poor appetite. In the study by Evans and his associates [11], appetite improved significantly among epoetin-treated patients. In a study by Lundin [12], 62 percent of dialysis patients rated their appetites as "poor" before the start of epoetin therapy. At the end of the study period, 91 percent of patients rated their appetites as "good." Patients ate more, increased their variety of foods, and reported that food tasted better. The large majority of studies assessing appetite found that more than 50 percent improved, and in some studies nearly all of the epoetin-treated ESRD patients improved [13, 14].

Sexual functioning is frequently impaired in ESRD patients. Men often report impotence and reduced sexual desire. Women are frequently infertile and have menstrual-cycle disorders. In the placebo-controlled Canadian multicenter trial [8], 20 of the 118 patients reported having problems of sexual functioning. Within eight weeks of epoetin therapy, this group reported more frequent and satisfying sexual relations. Several other studies support these findings [12].

ESRD patients may experience cognitive difficulties, such as confusion, impaired memory, or reductions in attention span. Using a variety of cognitive tests and measures of brain-wave response to stimuli, researchers have shown that epoetin therapy improves mental functioning [15].

Sleep disturbances are also common among patients with ESRD. These patients may nap frequently during the day. Many are unable to sleep well and do not awaken feeling rested. In a study of 329 dialysis patients, approximately 18 percent more patients reported waking up feeling fresh and rested always or almost always after receiving epoetin than before [11]. Deniston and her colleagues [16] also reported improvements in sleep and rest among 84 epoetin-treated patients compared with a non-epoetin control group. These findings are supported by several studies that assessed sleep habits among ESRD patients receiving epoetin therapy [12, 13].

Another dimension of quality of life adversely affected by renal anemia and improved with epoetin therapy is exercise capacity. Exercise capacity critically depends on the ability to increase oxygen supply to the body as physical activity is increased. In patients with ESRD, this capacity is frequently less than 50 percent of that of healthy individuals [17]. Diminished exercise capacity in this population is largely due to the reduced numbers of red blood cells. Epoetin, by stimulating the production of red blood cells and ameliorating renal anemia, markedly improves the exercise capacity of patients with ESRD [8, 11, 13, 14, 16]. This increase in endurance is expressed in patients' increased ability to work both in and outside of the home and to enjoy recreational activities.

The reversal of renal anemia and improvements in quality of life last only as long as epoetin therapy is continued. In a British study [14] of the effect of epoetin therapy, patients receiving epoetin showed a reversal of anemia and enhanced quality of life. At the end of the study period, when supplies of epoetin were withdrawn, the symptoms of renal anemia recurred, along with declines in quality of life.

Reimbursement Policies for Epoetin

According to the Social Security Amendments of 1972, all persons diagnosed with chronic, progressive kidney failure who are insured or eligible for benefits under Social Security, along with their spouses and dependent children, are entitled to Medicare ESRD benefits, regardless of age. In 1981, the Congress amended this legislation, making Medicare the secondary payer for the first twelve months of treatment for those beneficiaries also covered by their employer's group health insurance. The purpose of the 1981 amendment was to shift first-year treatment costs to private insurers and self-insuring employers [18].

Another piece of legislation—the Omnibus Budget Reconciliation Act of 1990 (OBRA-90)—changed the period of this secondary-payer provision from the first twelve months of treatment to the first eighteen months of Medicare entitlement. This extension affects an estimated 8,200 beneficiaries annually. It potentially lengthens the period of an employer's coverage by six to nine months, after which Medicare becomes the primary payer [18].

In 1991, nearly 150,000 ESRD patients received services through the Medicare ESRD program [1] at a cost of nearly $3.8 billion [19]. By the year 2000, an estimated 250,000 patients will be enrolled in the program [1].

When the Food and Drug Administration approved epoetin for the treatment of renal anemia in dialysis and predialysis patients in 1989, the HCFA announced that it would authorize payments for epoetin therapy. As mentioned earlier, Medicare reimburses providers 80 percent of allowable charges, which are set by Medicare. The remaining 20 percent must be paid by the patients or their secondary insurer. An estimated 70,000 to 80,000 persons with ESRD are covered by Medicare and receiving epoetin therapy [20]. Other dialysis patients may have low hematocrits but are not symptomatically anemic.

What follows is an illustration of how changes in epoetin reimbursement policies have affected patient treatment.

From June 1989 through December 1990, dialysis facilities were reimbursed for epoetin administration at a fixed-rate of either $40 for single doses up to 10,000 units or $70 for single doses over 10,000 units [19]. Reimbursement on this fixed-rate per-treatment basis created incentives to ration epoetin and to treat only those patients who would most likely benefit from low doses of the drug [19, 21].

According to Paul Eggers, Chief of the Evaluation Branch at HCFA, from November 1989 through December 1990, fewer than one-third of patients treated with epoetin reached target hematocrit levels [20]. Even among patients treated with epoetin for at least six months, fewer than half achieved hematocrit levels over 30 percent [21].

A national study of over 126,000 ESRD patients [19] found that prescriptions for epoetin during the first year after the drug's approval were related, in part, to factors such as race, gender, and dialysis setting. Women were more likely to receive epoetin than men, White patients more than Blacks, those aged below 35 years or over 65 years more than middle-aged patients, those undergoing in-center hemodialysis more than those who dialyze at home, and patients treated at for-profit dialysis centers more than those treated at not-for-profit centers. This study is important because it includes 93 percent of all U.S. dialysis patients and, because health insurance benefits were uniform across patients, the variability in health care coverage is eliminated. Its findings raise concerns about the possible relationship between access to care and non-clinical factors in health care decisions.

As of January 1991, Medicare changed the reimbursement system for epoetin. Under the new system, Medicare pays providers a dosage-linked fee of $11 for the first 1,000 units of epoetin administered, plus $1.10 for each increment of 100 units thereafter [22]. Under this system, there is no reimbursement ceiling on dosage levels. As before, however, Medicare will not reimburse providers for epoetin administered to ESRD patients whose hematocrit levels exceed 35 percent without written explanation by the physician. Most patients are able to carry out their daily activities with hematocrit values between 30 and 35 percent.

Under the dosage-linked reimbursement rate, the Medicare allowable charge per 1,000 units of epoetin dropped sharply, from $16.20 in December 1990 to approximately $11.63 in December 1991 [20]. Although this represents a substantial decline in the unit cost of epoetin, Medicare expenditures for epoetin have increased. In 1991, these costs were estimated at nearly $400 million annually. The increase in Medicare epoetin expenditures is due to an increase in the number of patients receiving epoetin and an increase in the mean dose from just under 2,700 units in November, 1989 to 3,450 units in December 1991. The percent of patients treated with epoetin reaching target hematocrit levels also increased, from approximately 18 percent in November 1989 to nearly 35 percent in December 1991 [20].

Medicare has made other changes in reimbursement policy that have expanded coverage for epoetin. As of July 1991, Medicare reimburses providers for epoetin administered at physicians' offices, licensed dialysis facilities, or patients' homes. Prior to this change, Medicare provided reimbursement only for epoetin administered at physicians' offices or licensed dialysis facilities. Medicare also extended coverage of epoetin for home dialysis patients who are competent to use the drug without direct medical supervision [22]. These changes in Medicare policy have eliminated the need for some home dialysis patients to travel to a clinic for epoetin therapy, although patients will still need periodic visits for monitoring.

J.D. may maximize the benefits of these policy changes by switching from in-center hemodialysis to at-home peritoneal dialysis. About 17 percent of ESRD patients are on peritoneal dialysis. This percentage is expected to rise to between 27 and 30 percent by 1996 [23]. Switching to peritoneal dialysis may be preferable for J.D. because it requires fewer dietary restrictions and enables patients more precisely to control their insulin and other medications. If she is able to switch from in-center hemodialysis to peritoneal dialysis, she also plans to begin to self-administer epoetin subcutaneously (that is, by injection into the tissue below the outer layer of the skin), just as she self-administers daily injections of insulin for her diabetes. She may require less epoetin per dose because smaller doses of subcutaneously administered epoetin may be as effective as larger intravenously administered doses (that is, by injection into a vein) [2].

Socioeconomic Consequences of Epoetin Therapy

Socioeconomic benefits may be assessed by balancing the extra costs of treating renal anemia with epoetin against the substantial gains in quality of life and levels of productivity at work or at home for both patients and their families.

Benefits of Epoetin Therapy: Epoetin versus Transfusions

Before the introduction of epoetin therapy, the standard treatment for severely anemic patients was blood transfusion. According to HCFA, annual Medicare expenditures for blood transfusions for ESRD patients totaled approximately $20 million before epoetin therapy. Since epoetin became the standard therapy for correcting ESRD anemia, Medicare expenditures for transfusions dropped 75 percent, to approximately $5 million annually [20]. This financial saving is negligible in comparison with the financial costs of epoetin. What is being sought here is the substantial improvement in quality of life from correction of the anemia.

Although the cost of epoetin therapy remains high relative to the savings in the cost of blood transfusions, epoetin does reduce the risks of exposure to hepatitis B and hepatitis non-A, non-B viruses and the human immunodeficiency virus (HIV) and of other transfusion-related illnesses, including iron overload and allergic reactions.

Before epoetin became available, J.D. had been hospitalized once for cardiac failure, which was related to her anemia. The cost for that hospitalization was more than the cost of a year's supply of epoetin. Since taking epoetin, she has not been hospitalized for any anemia-related illnesses.

Indirect benefits of epoetin therapy include enhanced quality of life and increased productivity both at home and at work. Patients who are able to care for themselves generally feel in greater control of their lives. They may utilize medical services more effectively, which could, in turn, help prevent the development of other conditions. Improved preventive measures might ultimately reduce morbidity and health care costs for this group.

Epoetin-treated patients report performing household tasks more effectively. By freeing family members from the demands of caring for the patient, quality of life for the entire family is often improved.

Barriers to Returning to Work

In the fall of 1991, J.D. felt well enough to resume working as an office manager, but she faced several barriers. Despite her qualifications and experience, many employers were unwilling to hire someone with chronic renal failure. Hiring an individual with a serious pre-existing medical condition is likely to raise the company's insurance costs or create problems in obtaining insurance. Furthermore, even though J.D. can self-dialyze at night and schedule evening appointments with her nephrologist, employers have been reluctant to take on the potential web of difficulties her health and her health care may present.

According to the General Accounting Office, OBRA-90 shifted an estimated $56 million in medical costs annually from Medicare to employers' health insurance plans. This may have adversely affected the ability of some ESRD patients to obtain or retain employment or employer-based health insurance. Among the 9 percent of ESRD patients who sought employment since becoming entitled to Medicare in May 1990, over one-third experienced at least one rejection for a job offering health coverage. Some patients reported that they were told their ESRD costs were the reason for their rejection, and others reported that they believed ESRD costs were a reason for their rejection—despite the fact that the Americans with Disability Act makes this kind of overt discrimination illegal. However, factors other than medical costs may be contributing to the loss of beneficiary jobs and health insurance coverage [*18*].

Fear of losing Social Security disability benefits prevents many patients from choosing to return to work. According to the Social Security Administration, if patients earn more than $500 per month for nine months (which need not be consecutive), they jeopardize benefits to themselves, their spouses, and dependent children [*24*]. Thus, although epoetin increases patients' work capacity by increasing both strength and endurance, many have been unable to realize their potential in the work force partly because of financial disincentives.

Conclusions

Since its approval by the Food and Drug Administration in 1989, epoetin has had widespread acceptance as the treatment of choice for renal anemia. Within the first year of approval, 52 percent of all dialysis patients and 60 percent of in-center dialysis patients covered by Medicare received epoetin [*19*].

Although patients with advanced renal failure continue to require dialysis to replace the filtering function of the kidneys, some of the symptoms previously thought to be part of the uremic syndrome may now be reversed by a correction of the patients' anemia. Reversal of anemia with epoetin has resulted in the elimination or reduction of the need for transfusion and dramatic improvements in patients' quality of life.

Between 70,000 and 80,000 Medicare ESRD patients receive epoetin therapy at an average cost of $6,000 per person annually. Although changes in Medicare reimbursement policy dramatically reduced the per-unit price of the drug, Medicare expenditures for epoetin therapy continue to rise because more people are receiving the drug at higher average doses. In 1991, estimated annual costs of epoetin were $400 million—nearly 7 percent of the Medicare ESRD budget.

Without Medicare coverage for epoetin therapy, many patients would not be able to afford the drug. Withdrawal of epoetin therapy results in a return to the anemic state and diminished quality of life.

Epoetin therapy has illuminated the distinction between patients' ability to work and barriers to employment. Changes in Medicare laws extending the period during which employer-based insurance carriers have primary responsibility for patients' medical costs may make it more difficult for ESRD patients to keep or find work.

For patients who are employed, epoetin may enable them to remain employed by eliminating the fatigue and other symptoms of renal anemia. These working patients may require more flexible dialysis schedules or may choose to dialyze at home. This will shift the demands on dialysis centers to provide treatment during evenings and weekends . It may also require centers to provide more patient education in self-care, home dialysis, self-administration of epoetin, and patient monitoring of their health status.

Epoetin therapy is still relatively new. Larger studies of ESRD patients treated with epoetin are under way. The multicenter National Cooperative Recombinant Human Erythropoietin Study will evaluate between 1,000 and 2,000 epoetin-treated chronic renal failure patients who are more broadly representative of the U.S. adult ESRD population [25]. Studies such as these will help to determine the larger impact of epoetin therapy on patients' mortality, morbidity, and quality of life.

Editors' Note

Relief of anemia by epoetin therapy in patients with ESRD causes measurable improvement in quality of life: patients report increased energy and exercise capacity, better sleep and appetite, more active social and sexual lives, and elimination of the need for transfusions. Because epoetin also may cause hypertension and blood clots, however, careful studies are required to measure the net benefits of treatment.

With improved well-being from continuous epoetin treatment, patients become more active, increasing demands for evening and weekend dialysis or for training for patient-conducted home dialysis. Thus one treatment success can change the demand for another.

Financial incentives embedded in the details of reimbursement policy also may alter the average effect of treatment of anemia or, given successful treatment of the anemia, the patient's return to work. The developments reported in this chapter emphasize once again the importance of searching for perverse effects of what may have seemed to be straightforward incentives. An example is the relation between insurance practices and the incentive to return to work rather than receive Social Security disability payments.

Experience rating, the adjustment of health insurance premiums of an employer based on the recent health care costs of that cadre of employees, creates a strong incentive to avoid hiring people who are likely to need health services, particularly ones that are expensive and chronic. That description fits the treatment of renal anemia with epoetin. Community rating, the adjustment of the employee's health insurance premiums based on the average expected health care costs of all beneficiaries in the community, would spread the financial risks of expensive services and thus mitigate the employer's incentives to avoid hiring those with pre-existing conditions or an increased risk of incurring high costs. Given the current regulations covering Social Security disability benefits, patients with ESRD on epoetin often fear losing their disability benefits if they respond to their epoetin-induced improvement in physical and mental performance by taking a job.

These problems can be addressed by community rating of health insurance premiums on the one hand, and some modification of the mechanism of the negative income tax on the other. The disability benefits would be structured so that increased income through employment would reduce the individual's disability benefit, but always at a rate that would provide the worker with a higher total income as a result of employment. Without some such interventions, the current system will continue to provide a treatment that greatly improves the capacity and function of recipients to lead normal, active lives while at the same time excluding them from the economy by enforcing rules that create perverse financial incentives to avoid employment.

PART D

Patient Empowerment

Many individuals who use medical services, and some who provide them, are seeking to negotiate a more equal and interactive patient-doctor relationship, a therapeutic alliance rather than cultivated dependency. Part of the motive force for this movement is ideological but some, at least, stems from the hypothesis that more participation and understanding *on the part of the patient* will yield better results *for the patient.* We examine this hypothesis for the perioperative period in the hospital.

The questions at issue are how preoperative education about pain control and postoperative control by the patient of administration of pain-relieving drugs affects the experience and the outcome of surgery. Many kinds of medications and cognitive-behavioral modifications, such as relaxation techniques, have been evaluated by carefully designed experiments with patients to find out, for the different therapies, whether the degree of pain relief is satisfactory, whether the treatment is safe, and which treatment is more appropriate for a given kind of patient. Of course, not all proposed techniques work, and those that do may not all work equally well.

Unfortunately, some patients and some health care workers who treat them are poorly informed about the desirability of proper pain control for good recovery. Consequently a substantial portion of patients have not received as much pain reduction as they should have or wish to have. Education for patients as well as medical personnel has been shown in many well-controlled studies to improve recovery after surgery. It is important to understand why patients often receive poor treatment when we have therapies that work.

8

The Control of Postoperative Pain

JANE C. BALLANTYNE, DANIEL B. CARR, JANICE ULMER,
ADA JACOX, AND DONNA MAHRENHOLZ

Introduction

In the fifty years that data on postoperative pain control, or analgesia, have been gathered, several surveys have documented that conventional treatment—intramuscular injections of standardized doses of morphine or meperidine (Demerol) "as needed"—leaves one-third to one-half of patients in moderate to severe pain during their postoperative stay [1]. Figure 8-1 illustrates the high frequency of failure in this area over a forty-year period. Today, we have potential remedies for our previous failures because we have a greater understanding of the neurophysiology and neuropharmacology of pain [2], new analgesic drugs and devices [3], and clinicians increasingly comfortable with the placement of catheters to target the delivery of drugs. Furthermore, though they will not be considered here, surgical techniques have also evolved rapidly to meet the public's and the medical profession's shared desire to avert needless suffering. (An example of one of these new techniques, laparoscopic surgery, is the subject of Chapter 3.) Finally, an emerging literature focusing on behavioral interventions suggests that these therapies can supplement drug treatments for moderate to severe pain and may suffice to control mild pain.

Two social forces—anxiety over the rising cost of health care and patients' desire to participate in choosing their own treatment—have increased concern for adequate pain relief after surgery. Of the more than 23 million operations now performed annually in the United States, a growing proportion are scheduled as same-day procedures. Postoperative hospital admission is increasingly restricted to patients who are undergo-

Percent of patients with
insufficient pain relief

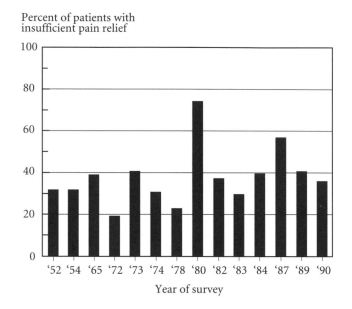

Figure 8-1. Percentage of patients experiencing insufficient pain relief or moderate to severe pain during conventional treatment. (Adapted with permission from Table 1 of the *Report of the Working Party on Pain after Surgery* by the Royal College of Surgeons [*1*].)

ing complex or extensive procedures, those who will suffer significant functional impairment requiring in-hospital recovery or close monitoring, or those who are frail because they are elderly or have coexisting diseases. The physiological and psychosocial risks associated with untreated pain are greatest in frail patients with other illnesses such as heart or lung disease, those undergoing major surgical procedures such as aortic surgery, and the very young or very old. Because of advances in surgical and anesthetic techniques, it is now common for such patients to undergo operations once dismissed as prohibitively risky. The clearest evidence for physiological benefits of effective pain control has emerged from studies of patients with limited physiological reserve undergoing major operations [4].

Increasing effort within the medical and nursing professions to improve postoperative pain control has led to position papers by surgical, anesthesiologic, and nursing organizations [5]. Dissemination of these and other guidelines in the popular press has informed patients and their families that "it doesn't have to hurt" after common operations once considered unavoidably painful; patients are now more likely to ask surgeons, anesthesiologists, and nurses about pain control before surgery, and the new awareness has encouraged the collaborative preparation of pain control plans. These plans feature technological advances, such as patient self-administration of analgesic drugs using miniaturized, programmable bedside pumps ("patient-controlled analgesia" [6], or PCA), along with deep breathing, relaxation, distraction exercises, or other behavioral techniques. These alternatives encourage patients not only to participate actively in their care but also teach them how to do it. In this chapter we will focus on PCA.

The following fictional vignette, a composite of many individual episodes, illustrates a typical example of the benefits of PCA. Professor W., now retired at age 76 after a distinguished teaching career, has been a heavy smoker all his life and takes medication daily to treat his pulmonary dysfunction. If he neglects to take his medicine, within a day he begins to wheeze and to feel short of breath. When his respiratory symptoms worsened recently, he had a chest x-ray, which disclosed a mass in his lung. He is referred to a thoracic surgeon, who schedules surgery for excision of this probable tumor. Preoperative testing of Professor W.'s pulmonary function reveals him to be at risk of becoming respirator-dependent after chest surgery.

Just before entering the operating room, Professor W. has a catheter (a small tube) placed next to his spine; local anesthetic is then injected through it so that his chest is numb before the operation begins. He awakens at the end of the operation with pain intensity at "2 of 10" arising

---

Policy Changes

Recent studies have shown that both patients and health care workers often do not understand the importance of pain control or the various means to achieve it. As a result, the National Cancer Institute and the Agency for Health Care Policy and Research have established new programs to promote improvements in the handling of cancer pain as well as acute pain. They have requested proposals for interventions that would improve the dissemination of modern guidelines for pain control and raise the quality of practice of analgesia.

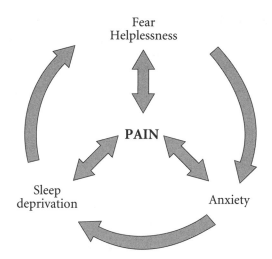

Figure 8-2. Pain, anxiety, and sleep deprivation reinforce one another. If pain persists unrelieved for several days, anger and depression also begin to contribute to the vicious circle as patients become demoralized and lose confidence in the ability (and motivation) of their medical attendants to relieve their pain. Sleeplessness compounds the problem. (Reproduced from Cousins and Phillips [7] with permission from Churchill Livingstone Inc.)

from the site of a chest drainage tube. Once or twice per day after surgery his pain starts to increase and he becomes anxious, but on these occasions he deliberately relaxes by letting his jaw go limp and finds that his distress subsides. After four days—during which no morphine has been used and doses of local anesthetic through the catheter have been slowly tapered— his chest drainage tube is removed, his pain declines to a level where he can control it using only "as needed" doses of an anti-inflammatory drug, he has his first postoperative bowel movement, and he resumes a normal diet. The catheter is then removed, and on the fifth postoperative day he is discharged home. Since the second postoperative day he has been alert and has used his time conversing on the telephone and completing a manuscript.

This case highlights the potential benefits of applying aggressive pain control in the postoperative period, particularly in the frail or "high-risk" patient in whom pain augments a vicious cycle of anxiety, helplessness, and sleep deprivation [7]. Figure 8-2 sums up the vicious circle of untreated pain. Although the humane goal of relieving unnecessary suffering is of course paramount, two broad lines of evidence from basic studies reinforce the value of aggressive pain control. First, it is now clear that the conscious perception of pain is just one of a group of linked negative physiological responses, such as changes in heart rate and blood pressure, triggered by tissue injury [2, 4]. These undesirable responses are evident even in patients under general anesthesia, in whom the conscious perception of pain does not exist. In the conscious patient unable to take a deep breath because it hurts too much, the already compromised pulmonary function that follows upper abdominal surgery can deteriorate further. Immobility due to the patient's desire to avoid pain on movement can increase the likelihood of postoperative deep venous thrombosis. In sum, "pain" is more than just suffering: it is intertwined with a number of key physiological responses, many of which are influenced by analgesia to the benefit of patient outcome.

A second body of evidence supporting the value of aggressive, even pre-emptive, pain control relates to the phenomenon of neural adaptation or "plasticity." Even a brief painful stimulus can induce long-lasting changes within nerves and the spinal cord, sensitizing them so that subsequent mild stimuli, not previously painful, become so [8].

Because acute pain is a malleable, dynamic process, and one that is linked to multiple physiologic responses, it is plausible that pain control may influence clinical outcome. On the other hand, pain therapy can cause its own problems: for example, the side effects of opiate drug therapy include respiratory depression and slowing of bowel transit time, and weakness and falling blood pressure may accompany spinal infusions of local anesthetics. Sufficient numbers of clinical trials have examined the effects of aggressive pain control on individual physiological parameters, such as vital capacity or length of stride, or postoperative morbidity, such as blood clots or pneumonia, to permit aggregation of these results according to quantitative statistical techniques. Methods for combining the results of several related studies to obtain more reliable conclusions are termed "meta-analytic techniques" (see Chapter 2). Outcome studies that go beyond measurements of physiological parameters to address other effects—such as mortality rates, costs, or length of stay in hospitals and intensive care units—have begun to appear [9].

In sum, several linked questions arise in recent assessments of the appropriateness of varied methods to achieve pain control:

1. To what extent does pain management alter postoperative morbidity?
2. What benefits (decreased cost of care, earlier discharge from hospital) result from reduced morbidity?
3. What are the costs of pain therapies—taking into account drugs, devices, physician and nursing time, and monitoring?

The remainder of this chapter will answer these questions for a pharmacological intervention (PCA) and selected cognitive-behavioral techniques. We also consider attempts to control pain through instruction and relaxation techniques before surgery only. The success of all the techniques surveyed herein hinges upon active participation of patients in their care.

Patient-Controlled Analgesia (PCA)

The constancy, in studies over the past fifty years, of the proportion of time that postoperative patients spend in moderate to severe pain suggests an underlying mathematical pattern in the sequence of time lags involved. A patient pushing the nurse call button must await the nurse's response and the completion of routine procedures before pain may be relieved: the nurse must assess the patient's pain, confirm the prescribed medicine and dose, locate the keys to the narcotic closet, draw up the medicine into a syringe and (if less than a complete ampoule of medicine is given) find a witness to watch him or her discard the unused portion of the controlled substance, and walk back to the patient's bedside before giving the intramuscular injection of the drug, which must be absorbed into the bloodstream before pain subsides. The cumulative survey data imply that these successive time lags lower the percentage of total time during which pain is well controlled to about 50 percent. When the patient cannot voice his or her discomfort, as may happen in the very young or very elderly, pain is likely to be well controlled during an even smaller percentage of time.

Because postoperative pain after major operations lasts for days while the effect of any common pain medication only lasts for hours, the standard approach to pain relief may be likened to driving cross-country until the gas tank is empty, then pushing one's car in search of the next gas station, then repeating this cycle for a week! In both instances an anticipatory approach to an inevitable shortfall minimizes the time spent dealing with "refueling." Even when an anticipatory approach has not been taken, reducing the time lag between a patient's perception of discomfort and treatment of this discomfort will diminish average pain intensity. This reduction in time lag is central to the idea of PCA, as, too, is the enhanced degree of control that patients have over their own therapy.

Although patients placed on PCA control the timing of their own doses of analgesic drug, the magnitude of each dose, the minimal "lockout" time between successive possible dosings, the maximum dose per unit time, and other parameters are set by the physician or nurse. By pushing a button, patients can self-administer intravenous doses of analgesic drug whenever they feel it is necessary—limited only by the pre-set parameters. The method has obvious advantages, particularly to patients. The patient does not have to wait for the nurse's response and delivery of the drug, nor for an intramuscular dose to be systemically absorbed. Because of the ease of administering each injection, small and frequent doses can be given, so that peaks and troughs in serum drug levels are avoided. The method has become very popular with patients, physicians, and nurses [10].

Many claims have been made for PCA—that it produces superior analgesia, that overall analgesic usage is less, that side effects are minimized, and that recovery from surgery is accelerated because of early return to full mobility and more comfortable breathing. We have used meta-analyses (see Chapter 2) to evaluate analgesic efficacy, overall analgesic usage, and the satisfaction of patients with PCA in comparison with conventional therapy [9]. We have also analyzed length of hospital stay associated with the two methods and compared side effects in the two treatment groups.

Conventional therapy itself is effective in reducing pain, particularly when patients receive it during a controlled trial, in which their need for pain medicine is apt to be assessed more intensively than usual. The difference between pain intensity experienced during PCA versus conventional therapy in controlled trials is about 6 points on a scale of 0 to 100, spanning no pain (0 on the scale) to pain that is unbearable (100 on the scale). The advantage of PCA is that it avoids the excesses and shortfalls of conventional, nurse-applied analgesics. Patients using PCA regulate their drug delivery to avoid deep analgesia, with its associated sedation, as they prefer to remain alert while keeping their pain within tolerable limits [11]. Figure 8-3 displays the frequency (indicated by the height of the blocks) of different levels of sedation and pain observed in patients using PCA following a surgical operation. Most patients have a desirable state of comfort along with a high level of alertness.

To sum up, PCA is superior to conventional therapy in controlling pain.

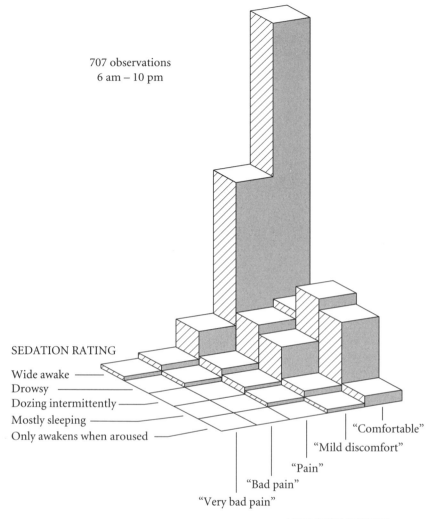

707 observations
6 am – 10 pm

SEDATION RATING

Wide awake
Drowsy
Dozing intermittently
Mostly sleeping
Only awakens when aroused

"Comfortable"
"Mild discomfort"
"Pain"
"Bad pain"
"Very bad pain"

ANALGESIA RATING

Figure 8-3. Concurrent analgesia and sedation ratings made during normal waking hours (6:00 A.M.–10:00 P.M.) in a group of 50 patients using PCA following elective surgery (laparotomy). The majority of observations indicate a state of analgesia with minimal sedation. Near-optimal drug titration appears to be effectively accomplished with PCA. (Reproduced from Bennett [*11*] with permission from Blackwell Scientific Publications Ltd.)

Although no more opioid drug is used, patients prefer PCA to conventional therapy, and PCA can be recommended for these reasons alone. The miniaturization and computer control of instruments have made PCA feasible for widespread use.

Nonpharmacologic Interventions

Nonpharmacologic approaches to pain management are increasingly recognized as legitimate interventions for pain relief. Melzack and Wall [12] hypothesized almost three decades ago that higher brain centers can influence the passage of pain signals through the spinal cord. Yet it was not until specific anatomical circuits and mechanisms were demonstrated in research laboratories that a scientific basis for the power of the mind to influence the body emerged. Scientists now believe that pathways that descend to the spinal cord from areas of the brain responsible for thought and emotion are able to modulate pain signals. As research continues to unravel the intricate nature of the body's pain response systems, clinicians are beginning to demonstrate the effectiveness of cognitive-behavioral interventions. Cognitive-behavioral interventions provide patients with more information about their pain and then enable them take an active part in its assessment and control. The goals of therapy are to alter pain perception, to alter pain behavior, and to provide a greater sense of control over pain.

Devine [13] refers to these interventions collectively as "psychoeducational" interventions. Other researchers classify psychoeducational interventions according to whether they affect the way one thinks, the way one behaves, or both (these are cognitive, behavioral, or cognitive-behavioral interventions). Within each class of interventions a variety of patient responses can be observed or taught. Most of us have some strategy that we use automatically when we are confronted with pain or distress. For example, during a dental appointment we might count ceiling tiles or talk encouragingly to ourselves ("the pain is not that bad," "it will soon be over"). These are cognitive strategies, distraction (the tile counting) and positive self-statement.

Health professionals use these and other strategies to promote the ability of the mind to modify the body's responses to pain. Such an approach empowers patients by encouraging them to participate in their care and by building upon their innate coping strengths. Advantages of cognitive-behavioral strategies are that, once learned, they can be used in any place, at any time. They can also be applied to other distressing life experiences. When used to manage pain, these interventions are best individualized to meet the needs and personal characteristics of the person seeking relief.

The discussion that follows is limited to two specific types of strategy: preoperative teaching and relaxation training. These were selected because they are two of the most commonly used and studied cognitive-behavioral interventions for the management of postoperative pain.

Preoperative Teaching

Intuitively, it would seem that instructing patients before surgery how to decrease the pain of postoperative coughing, deep breathing, turning, and ambulation would better prepare them to meet the challenges of a surgical experience. Knowing what to expect prepares patients for surgery by

---

The Benefits of Education in Recovery from Surgery

Research in the 1980s (Devine and Cook, 1983, 1986) indicated that brief patient education prior to surgery about what to expect during recovery speeded the patient's release from the hospital. Since then great changes in the management of surgery have reduced hospital stays considerably. In a recent meta-analysis, Devine (1992) showed that education about the course of recovery from surgery, usually delivered by registered nurses, improved recovery, reduced pain, reduced psychological distress, and reduced length of hospital stay. All these improvements were of the order of magnitude of four-tenths of a standard deviation. These effects hold up well across kinds of hospital and a variety of kinds of surgery.

Devine, E. C., and T. D. Cook. 1983. A meta-analytic review of psycho-educational interventions on length of hospital stay. *Nursing Research* 32:267–274.

———— 1986. Clinical and cost relevant effects of psychoeducational interventions with surgical patients: A meta-analysis. *Research in Nursing and Health* 9:89–105.

Devine, E. C. 1992. Effects of psychoeducational care with adult surgical patients: A theory-probing meta-analysis of intervention studies. In T. D. Cook et al., eds. *Meta-Analysis for Explanation: A Casebook*, 35–82. New York: Russell Sage Foundation.

---

removing uncertainty and feelings of helplessness [14]. Knowing what discomforts they will feel, and what they can do to aid recovery, provides patients with a sense of a normal recovery. Patients who have learned how to use a pain scale have a means to communicate pain and a yardstick to gauge the effectiveness of pain relief. Each of these measures provides patients with a sense of control.

For the reasons discussed in Chapter 2, we performed three meta-analyses on a collection of fourteen papers to evaluate the effects of preoperative teaching on self-reports of pain, analgesic use, and length of hospital stay [15]. The first analysis found no differences in levels of pain between experimental and control subjects. The second analysis found that patients given preoperative teaching used less opioid analgesic medication than control subjects. And the third analysis concluded that patients who received an educational intervention had shorter hospital stays.

Relaxation

One approach clinicians have used to alleviate pain and anxiety in postoperative patients is to teach them a cognitive-behavioral intervention aimed at promoting relaxation. Relaxation is the most widely studied cognitive-behavioral approach to postoperative pain management. The goal of relaxation therapy is to instill a sense of control over pain and thus modify the way a person thinks about and reacts to pain. Various relaxation techniques may employ a quiet environment; a comfortable position; mental "exercises" to reduce distracting thoughts; a script with phrasing that encourages a passive attitude; repetition and practice of certain behaviors; conscious acts that condition a relaxation response, such as a yawn or deep breath; and options for patient control [16].

Meta-analysis of fifteen papers was used to evaluate the effects of relaxation interventions on the same measures as above: pain intensity, analgesic use, and length of hospital stay [15]. The analyses found that patients who were taught a relaxation exercise reported less pain and required significantly less opioid analgesics than subjects who received "usual care." In this set of papers only four recorded data on hospital length of stay; no reliable differences were found.

To sum up, these results suggest that, just as with preoperative education about the course of surgical recovery, patients benefit when they are taught a relaxation exercise before surgery. Each of the studies included in this analysis concerned a relatively simple relaxation procedure or script, and usually only a single patient contact was required to teach the intervention. The amount of professional time devoted to teaching averaged 15 minutes or less. Once taught, patients were able to use the relaxation exercise independently and without coaching.

The findings from studies that evaluated the efficacy of simple relaxation, imagery, and music-assisted relaxation suggest that these interventions may be effective in decreasing self-reported pain and analgesic use. Other evidence, not reviewed here, suggests that relatively simple cognitive-behavioral interventions are as effective as more complex ones.

Costs

The cost of conventional analgesic therapy for postoperative patients is often disregarded, but it is not negligible. Although all postoperative patients should be under observation, special monitoring is not normally provided when conventional therapy is used. As we have described, however, nursing time is used every time an injection is needed. Jackson has done a detailed cost analysis assessing PCA versus intramuscular analgesia [*17*]. She estimates that the average number of injections needed by a cholecystectomy patient in the first 48 hours postoperatively is 10. The nursing procedure for intramuscular injections was timed and found to take an average of 15 minutes per injection. (Only one nurse was needed to prepare and administer injections in this study, though sometimes two are required.) At $0.22 per minute, the nursing cost was $33 for 10 injections.

Patient-controlled analgesia has the advantage that once the infusion pump is charged and its parameters set, the patients administer their own doses. Jackson also assesses the cost of PCA. The nursing procedure for PCA was timed. When the patient arrived on the ward, the nurse initiated the PCA procedure, which took an average of 5 minutes. An additional 25 minutes was included in the total cost for subsequent charting of dosages and changing syringes. For cholecystectomy, PCA is needed for an average of 48 hours. Total nursing time used during the 48 hours is 30 minutes—a cost of $6.60 for nursing time. Ready has also presented survey data based on his and colleagues' experience in the Seattle area [*18*]. In his institution, 24 nurses were asked to estimate time requirements to provide postoperative analgesia using conventional intramuscular injections or PCA. The times estimated for each shift were 39 minutes with conventional therapy versus 28 minutes with PCA. With 11 minutes saved per shift, for three shifts per day, Ready concluded that 33 nurse-minutes per day were saved when PCA was used in place of conventional postoperative medication. The reduced cost of nursing time during PCA use is offset by the cost of the device. A PCA pump costs between two and three thousand dollars, though prices are decreasing. Ready has published preliminary data to suggest that a patient charge of $37.50 per day will more than offset hospital costs of leasing a PCA pump.

Two important factors must also be taken into account in an evaluation of the cost of pharmacologic pain therapy: the need and cost of providing monitoring, and the cost benefit from reducing postoperative morbidity. The provision of monitoring for patients being treated for pain is of the utmost importance, not only in detecting side effects and complications but also in ensuring adequate analgesia. Monitoring does not necessarily require the use of expensive apparatus, such as those required for automated blood pressure measurement, electrocardiography, and pulse oximetry. In fact, while such devices are useful adjuncts to monitoring, it is dangerous to rely on them alone. With or without the aid of monitoring equipment, the cost of monitoring is a major component of the overall cost of pain therapy. Thus, the costs of PCA are incompletely studied at present and require further analyses of cost savings and other benefits of these interventions.

Conclusions

Although studies of clinical correlates of postoperative pain treatment are still comparatively few, it is clear that PCA and cognitive-behavioral methods allow for improved pain control compared to conventional "as-needed" dosing regimens. For certain patient subgroups, undesirable clinical outcomes, such as pulmonary dysfunction or thromboembolism, are reduced during aggressive pain control, although the improvement in clinical outcome is not always clearly correlated with reductions in pain intensity. Further work in this field must evaluate not only innovative technologies but also the economics and feasibility of different organizational models to achieve postoperative pain control in an era of increasingly stringent health care reimbursement policies.

The development of modern techniques of pain relief has been followed by their broad application in the postoperative setting. The new techniques allow patients to control their pain quickly and effectively and thus have meshed well with patients' wishes for "empowerment" in their care and the decisions surrounding it. In the instance of pain relief (as for other circumstances), shifting more control to patients and fostering their participation in their own care have raised their levels of postoperative comfort and satisfaction with their treatment.

Editors' Note

Carefully controlled studies have shown that patients' recovery from surgical operations improves when their pain is kept under control. Patients, nurses, and physicians often need training in this matter—not only does a surgical procedure not have to hurt so much, but hurting delays recovery. Conventional dispensing of pain medication "as needed" leaves one-third to one-half of patients with inadequate pain control at least part of the time.

The poor record of conventional analgesia may seem paradoxical, given that successful technologies are available, but several causes can be identified. First, in conventional treatment the other obligations of nurses and the need for security in handling pain-relieving drugs lead to substantial delays between the moment the patient requests relief and administration of the analgesic. Second, both health care workers and patients often have exaggerated impressions about the dangers of addiction from postoperative medications. Third, in the medical system as a whole, knowledge of modern techniques of handling pain is not well disseminated. Fourth, many physicians have not been informed of the benefits of pain relief to recovery.

Determining what pain-relief techniques in what modes of administration are effective requires well-controlled studies. These investigations also produce information about undesirable effects on respiration, bowel function, and blood pressure. Patient-controlled anesthesia promotes patient satisfaction, avoids sedation while using the same amount of medication, and achieves better control because the "peaks and troughs" of pain are avoided. More generally, effective preoperative education and pain control reduce hospital length of stay.

PART E

Monitoring and Delivering Care

The efforts to develop powerful medicines for the prevention or treatment of serious acute and chronic diseases make up some of the most exciting chapters in the history of modern medicine. The battle against infectious diseases such as measles has provided many dramatic examples. As related in this section, a measles vaccine virtually eliminated measles and its complications of death, mental retardation, and deafness, but the disease rebounded as the rates of infant immunization were allowed to fall. Grouped with this case study is a success story concerning a disease less alarming than an outbreak of measles but one that has severe consequences for many Americans. Called the "silent killer," hypertension is responsible for a large number of strokes and heart attacks every year, especially among Blacks. A concerted campaign to identify hypertension among Blacks, lower the barriers that impede their access to health care, and bring them into effective treatment has largely eliminated the differential in successful treatment between Blacks and Whites.

These two cases share a common feature: both measles and hypertension require multipronged social intervention for their control. Our stumbling progress with respect to measles and our relative programmatic successes with respect to hypertension offer a variety of important lessons about delivering and monitoring health services across a population.

9

Immunization against Measles

DONALD N. MEDEARIS, JR.

The History and Societal Impact of Measles

To call measles one of the usual childhood diseases is to trivialize a serious illness. Its most frequent manifestations—sneezing, coughing, conjunctivitis, fever, and rash lasting several days—are so characteristic that an observer can reliably make its diagnosis. It is a highly contagious viral infection with a very high disease-infection ratio; that is, 90 percent of those who are exposed and are not immune become infected, and 90 percent of those infected manifest disease. Thus, without immunization, almost all of each year's newborn population will get the disease sometime during infancy or childhood.

Some of the more serious complications of measles are pneumonia, croup, diarrhea, and inflammation of the brain or encephalitis (sometimes followed by mental retardation); it can also be fatal. In immunocompromised individuals, such as those with leukemia or AIDS or those taking immunosuppressive drugs to help transplanted organs survive, the virus may continue to multiply as a result of the absence of cell-bound immunity. In such patients, two severe complications may occur: a rare kind of pneumonia called giant-cell pneumonitis, which may proceed without the usual rash and is often fatal, and encephalitis [1, 2].

The disease has been written about since the seventh century. It was distinguished from smallpox by the Arabian physician Rhazes in the tenth century; its clinical manifestations were described more precisely by the English physician Thomas Sydenham in the seventeenth century; and it was shown to be transmissible in the eighteenth century by Sir Everard Home, who took the blood of one patient and by inoculating it into another induced measles [1]. It has been stated that when societies were able to maintain cities of several hundred thousand population, measles became endemic. The result was that measles occurred in young children and the surviving adult population came to be comprised of immune individuals. When Europeans come to the New World from such cities and brought measles to the native populations, who had never been exposed to the disease, the result was devastating. Thirty thousand Amazon Indians died in an epidemic in 1749 [3]. The disease has been devastating in military populations too: during the Civil War, 75,000 soldiers had measles and 5,000 died, and 2,000 soldiers died of the 90,000 who developed measles in World War I [3].

Measles virus has no animal reservoir. The infection is transmitted person to person by large droplets produced by sneezing or coughing. Before immunization became available, the usual number of cases of measles reported each year in the United States was about 500,000. In all probability, however, the actual number of cases was the same as that year's cohort of toddler-aged children (probably several million), so infectious is this agent. Of every 1,000 of those who contract the disease, 38 will develop pneumonia, bronchitis, or croup; 25 will develop otitis media; 12 will be hospitalized; and 1 will develop encephalitis (and of those with encephalitis a number will become mentally retarded).

The risk of death from measles is 1 in 10,000 [3]. When death occurs during the acute phase of the disease in children, it is usually the result of pneumonia, which may be a secondary bacterial infection. In older individuals, death is more often the result of encephalitis. Fortunately, one severe complication is also one of the rarest. Subacute sclerosing panencephalitis (SSPE), a chronic, progressive, and debilitating disease of the central nervous system, becomes manifest about 8 years after the initial episode of measles. It appears to be the result (at least in part) of the failure of the virus to stimulate an immune response in the patient, with the consequence that a persistent infection of the central nervous system is established. It occurs after fewer than 1 of every 100,000 cases of measles in otherwise normal individuals.

The measles virus was isolated and grown in tissue culture by Enders and Peebles in the 1950s. Serial passage of the virus through tissue culture reduced its virulence for humans to the point where it could safely be used as a live-virus, anti-measles vaccine. That is, the severity of the disease caused by the attenuated virus was much reduced but stimulated produc-

Vitamin A Supplementation and Child Mortality

Two sets of randomized trials have been examined to assess the benefit of vitamin A supplementation for reducing the death rate in children. One set of studies included the administration of vitamin A to hospitalized measles patients in Capetown, Durban, Tanzania, and London, England. A meta-analysis of these four studies showed that the supplementation cut the death rate by more than half, from over 9 percent to less than 4 percent.

The second set consisted of community studies carried out in the field. In six communities, randomly chosen villages, districts, or households were assigned to treatment groups, which would receive vitamin A supplementation, or to control groups. The sites were Sarlahi and Jumia in Nepal, an area in northern Sudan, Aceh in Indonesia, and Tamil Nadu and Hyderabad in India. In the meta-analysis, averaging across the six randomized studies, the treated groups were found to have about 25 percent lower death rates than the control groups. The death rates in children aged 6–72 months were over 12 per 1,000 in the control groups. The communities differed in the effectiveness of the treatment, with northern Sudan and Hyderabad showing no benefit but the other four communities showing considerable benefit, all of similar magnitudes.

Only four of the six studies reported cause of death, but in those that did diarrhea was identified as the cause of half of the deaths. The supplement of vitamin A was associated with a 30 percent reduction in such deaths.

Because vitamin A deficiency is widespread in developing countries, supplementation appears valuable. For measles patients it seems wise whether vitamin A deficiency is present or not.

Fawzi, W. W., et al. 1993. Vitamin A supplementation and child mortality. *Journal of the American Medical Association* 269:898–903.

tion by the patient of an antibody response to the natural measles virus. Once stimulated, this antibody response would provide immunity against the disease if the patient were ever exposed to the natural, virulent form of the virus.

In contrast to the dramatic reduction in the frequency of measles brought about by measles vaccination in developed countries, measles continues to take a tragic toll on the children of the less developed countries of the world. There, millions of children die each year as a result of measles. Death occurs most frequently as a result of pneumonia or diarrhea in these patients, who so often are malnourished or afflicted with other debilitating conditions.

The extent of the economic burden of measles to our society can be estimated from the morbidity and mortality figures provided above: given that there were approximately 4,000,000 cases per year and that the annual cost was $670,000,000, an estimate can be made that the annual cost per 10,000 cases would be about $1,675,000 in 1985 dollars [2]. We will have more to say on this topic in the section below on cost-effectiveness.

Therapeutic Interventions

Prior to the advent of measles immunization, most adults had had measles and as a result had antibodies to measles. Thus pools of gamma globulin (a type of protein found in the blood) containing antibody to measles could be obtained from these adults. Gamma globulin is effective in preventing disease, though its effect is transient. For example, the intramuscular administration of the immunoglobulin within six days of a recognized exposure prevented measles in 80 percent of the recipients. Of those in whom the disease was not prevented, only a small percentage had typical measles with the usual frequency of complications. In the others, the disease was much more mild. (See reference [2] for a more detailed discussion of measles vaccinations.)

Intravenous gamma globulin is now available for administration to individuals who require repeated doses of such preparations because of their continuing immunodeficient state; it will prevent or ameliorate measles. This is an important preventive modality because of the otherwise devastating effects that measles may have in the patient whose immune system is compromised as a result of AIDs, chemotherapy for cancer, or medications given for organ transplantation. A number of other therapies have been tried, including antiviral agents such as ribavirin and biologic agents such as interferon and thymic humoral factor, but none have proved to be effective. Traditional antibiotics help in treating or ameliorating bacterial complications of measles, including bacterial pneumonia, but do not alter the measles infection itself.

A significant beneficial effect of vitamin A has been demonstrated in patients from countries in which vitamin deficiencies are common. In a study in Africa, Hussey and Klein [4] treated 92 infants with measles with vitamin A and 97 with an identical-appearing placebo. The two groups were similar, and vitamin A treatment was begun within a few days of the onset of rash. Only 2 of the 92 in the treated group died; in contrast, of the 97 in the placebo group, 10 died. The frequency of croup, the duration of pneumonia and diarrhea, the length of hospitalization, and the frequency of admission to the intensive care unit were all reduced in the vitamin A treatment group. Similar findings have been made recently in the United States [5].

Vaccine: Its Development and Use

Testing the first live-virus vaccine revealed that, in contrast to natural measles, which caused a fever greater than 103°F in 96 percent of the cases and a rash in all, only 30 percent of vaccine recipients developed that degree of fever and only 50 percent developed rash. Additional passages of the virus through tissue culture, and thus further attenuation of it, reduced the frequency of fever to 5–15 percent and of rash to about 5 percent. The vaccine was found effective when administered alone or combined with the other vaccines administered to children. Combining vaccines reduces cost, effort, and discomfort. In the United States the most commonly used vaccine is one which contains measles, mumps, and rubella viruses, all of which are attenuated live-virus vaccines. This practice has not resulted in a decreased extent or frequency of antibody response or protection; and it has not been associated with increased frequency or severity of side effects.

Use of the vaccine as recommended induces an antibody response and its associated immunity in 95 percent of recipients. In the population, 2–5 percent fail to respond to a vaccine that apparently is potent. The cause of failure to respond is unknown; no genetic factors have been found. The majority of all data accumulated indicate that development of antibodies after a single dose of live-virus vaccine properly administered to an appropriate recipient is associated with lifelong protection.

Although the vaccine is a live virus, its attenuation is such that it has not been shown to spread from one individual to another, as live-poliovirus vaccine may.

The side effects of vaccine administration are infrequent and mild. The fever is much less than is seen in measles unmodified by pre-existing immunity, as is the duration and nature of the rash. The frequency of encephalitis after measles vaccine is less than 1 in 1,000,000. Other side effects have been reported with very much lower frequency than with natural measles.

Few individuals have contraindications to receiving live measles-virus vaccine. Individuals with AIDS should not be vaccinated with attenuated live-virus vaccine except in those countries where HIV infection, the cause of AIDS, is very common. Measles can be devastating in children with HIV infection, but the available data indicate that the vaccine, on balance, is beneficial in HIV-infected children. Many children with HIV infection, even those with symptoms, have been vaccinated without serious adverse consequences. In them, the antibody response may be less; the reduced immune response is associated with lower counts of the white blood cells that are crucial to normal immunity.

Two factors can reduce the effectiveness of measles vaccine. The presence of maternal antibody to measles in an infant can prevent or reduce the multiplication of the virus in the vaccine so that the viral mass produced in the infant is not sufficent to stimulate an adequate immune response. When 9-month-old (or younger) infants were vaccinated, a large proportion of them failed to develop long-lasting immunity. When exposed to the virus later, these individuals were not protected and got measles. Accordingly, studies were carried out to determine when in infancy it is best to administer live attenuated measles virus vaccine. In some countries with high rates of measles in infants, it is recommended that the vaccine be administered at 6 months of age, and again at 15 months of age. Where infants have low rates of measles, vaccine should be given at 15 months of age and then on entry to middle school or junior high school.

Live attenuated measles virus vaccine, like other viral vaccines, must be preserved by refrigeration. It quickly loses potency at room temperature; this effect of temperature is the cause of some vaccine failures.

Vaccination: Its Cost-Effectiveness

Attenuated measles virus vaccine has been extremely effective; the infrequent side effects and occasional apparent vaccine failures have been of little public health importance. The vaccine was licensed in 1963 and its effect was dramatic. There were about 450,000 cases of measles in 1964, but only 250,000 in 1965. In 1986 there were 6,282 cases; that is a reduction of almost 99 percent [6] from the estimated incidence prior to 1963, a reduction of 99.8 percent from the earlier 4 million cases per year.

Recognizing that the vaccine had been extremely effective, Bloch and co-authors [3] calculated the health and resource benefits that have accrued through its use in the United States from 1963 through 1982. They wrote that more than 52,000,000 cases of measles were averted, and that over 5,000 lives had been saved. More than 17,000 cases of mental retardation were avoided and 1.5 million years of normal, productive life had been won. Approximately 27 million doctor visits were saved, and almost 3 million hospital days avoided. They estimated that the savings amounted to $5 billion!

In two studies that addressed the issue of the cost-effectiveness of giving measles vaccine alone, each dollar spent saved ten dollars in health care costs and productivity [6].

The total cost of vaccinating a child against diphtheria, pertussis, tetanus, poliomyelitis, measles, mumps, rubella and *Haemophilus influenzae* type B meningitis via public sector programs is $82.90; in the private sector it is somewhat more than $100. With costs taken into account, the net savings for one year, 1981, from the overall program of multiple immunizations were estimated to be $700 million by Koplan and White; the estimate by Bloch and colleagues for that year was $630 million [3].

The Measles Outbreaks of 1989 and 1990

In 1978 an effort to eradicate measles was begun, and in 1983 a record low number of measles cases was reported, 1,497. Then, suddenly and unexpectedly, there was a sevenfold increase in reported measles cases from a median incidence of 1.3 cases/100,000 population for the years 1981–1988 to 7.3 in 1989 and 11.2 in 1990 [7]. The United States had 18,193 cases in 1989 and 27,786 reported cases in 1990 [7]. The greatest increase was in those under 5 years of age; 48 percent of the reported cases in 1990 were in that group, whereas in the period 1980–1988 only 29 percent of the cases were in children that young. The incidence was highest in Blacks and Hispanics [7]. Of all measles cases, 47 percent reported in 1990 were associated with but 5 outbreaks; the majority of cases in 1989 and 1990 were in the inner cities of large metropolitan areas [6]. During the 1980s, 53.9 percent of the nation's 3,137 counties reported no cases of measles. Only 17 counties reported cases in each of the ten years 1980 through 1989. These counties had higher median populations and population densities, and a higher percentage of Hispanic and Black populations [8]. Thus, the 1989 and 1990 outbreaks were characterized by the disproportionate occurrence of measles in young Black and Hispanic children who were living in the inner cities of large metropolitan areas and who should have been vaccinated but who had not been.

Several authors have found that even those pre-schoolers who had access to health care were the victims of lost opportunities for vaccination. In Rochester, New York, for example, 82 percent of 422 children under 36 months of age had missed an opportunity to receive an immunization. Indeed, on average, each child missed 7.2 opportunities to be immunized [9].

Other studies also indicated that these outbreaks were due mostly to a failure to vaccinate. Hinman [10] reported that in Chicago, 80 percent of the pupils in predominantly White, middle-class schools had received measles vaccine by their second birthday, whereas only 50 percent of the students in predominantly Black or Hispanic schools had received measles vaccine by their second birthday. Moreover, for 25 percent of the students in predominantly Black or Hispanic schools, vaccine administration was delayed until after 4 years of age; in contrast, this delay was infrequent in predominantly White schools. Not surprisingly, measles attack rates correlated inversely with the immunization rates.

Hinman listed several factors associated with the failure to receive vaccine. Children were uninsured, eligible for Medicaid but unenrolled, and impeded by geographic, ethnic, and administrative factors. He said their parents might have been unaware of the importance of immunization; and, he wrote, "We have no comprehensive system of ensuring or tracking preventive health services for children in this country" [10].

There are, of course, other factors that may have contributed to the occurrence of these outbreaks. Were the outbreaks due to a failure of the vaccine to protect? Was there a new, more virulent strain of measles abroad? A study in California revealed that the incidence of measles among children in households with an initial case of measles was 78 percent in unvaccinated children 1–5 years old but only 4 percent in those who had been vaccinated [11]. The vaccine was still highly effective, therefore, and the measles virus causing these outbreaks appeared to be unchanged. Other observations indicated that many of the infants and children who got measles had been born to young mothers. These mothers may have been immune to measles as a result of having received measles vaccine. The antibody induced by the vaccine and present during the gestation of the child who got measles may have been different from the antibody produced by mothers who had had natural measles, or present in lower concentrations. If so, then the amount of antibody to measles that crossed the placenta from mother to fetus in utero may have been less protective [12]. This possibility has not been established, but it should be explored.

Lessons for the Future

After reviewing the available data, the National Vaccine Advisory Committee [13] concluded that the principal cause for the marked increase in measles in the United States in 1989–1990 was the failure to provide vaccine to vulnerable children on schedule. It went on to assert that the primary reasons for that failure existed within our health care system. It emphasized that ideally immunization should be given as a part of a comprehensive child health program. The committee recognized that a comprehensive child health program will not be established in the immediate future but that several recommendations should be acted on in the interim.

It noted the lack of national coordination of vaccine programs and of information on federal expeditures on immunization programs, even though half of the vaccines given children are administered in the public sector and federal programs provide the funds to purchase about one-half of these vaccines. The committee believed that children were not being vaccinated in part because the public had not been made sufficiently aware of the importance and value of immunization and as a result didn't demand immunization. Fragmentation of responsibility for programs of preventive care means that no one is fully accountable for the burden of preventable illness and for monitoring its prevalence. Fragmentation of the U.S. health care budget means that the dollar savings due to childhood immunizations are overlooked.

In 1990 the CDC surveyed the 54 largest immunization projects in an attempt to determine what barriers to immunization were felt to exist [14]. Twenty-seven project leaders identified no barriers. The remaining 27 identified the following barriers: that immunizations were available only by appointment (93 percent of 27 projects); that physical examinations were required prior to immunization (56 percent); that a physician referral was required (41 percent); that prior enrollment in the well-baby clinic was required (37 percent); and, lastly, 22 percent stated that administrative fees were a barrier. Other problems included insufficient clinical personnel,

---

The Children's Vaccine Initiative

The Children's Vaccine Initiative has identified six goals for improving the delivery of immunization and health care.

1. Reduce the number of contacts required to fully immunize a child. UNICEF estimates that today it takes more than 500 million separate contacts annually to achieve current levels of immunization against six diseases.
2. Reduce dependence on refrigeration. The cold chain costs as much as the vaccines themselves.
3. Reduce the use of needles, syringes, and sterilization equipment, which are expensive and pose a threat for the transmission of hepatitis B and HIV.
4. Achieve the protection offered by vaccines at an earlier age and make it last longer.
5. Develop new vaccines that permit the prevention of at least another dozen diseases that persist as major hazards to children.
6. Achieve all these advances and improvements in ways that are affordable to developing countries and contributing donors.

Source: Quoted from page 5 of P. Freeman and A. Robbins, "Introduction: Vaccine technologies and public health, 1994," *International Journal of Technology Assessment in Health Care,* 10:1–6. Copyright © 1994 Cambridge University Press. Reprinted with the permission of Cambridge University Press.

inadequate or inconvenient clinic hours, too few or inconvenient clinic locations, and language and cultural problems. It was notable that unavailability of the vaccine itself was not reported as a major problem.

In the private sector, obstacles included the fact that private physicians passed the high cost of vaccine on to their patients. The cost of measles, mumps, and rubella vaccine according to the federal contract price is $15.33; the catalogue price is $25.29 [13]. These increased prices are passed on to the patient, but many of their health insurers do not cover immunizations. Employment-based plans with conventional health insurance covered only 45 percent of instances of immunization; preferred provider plans, 62 percent; health maintenance organizations, 98 percent.

The unavailability of health care of any kind would, of course, be associated with the failure to be able to obtain immunization. In 1988, Black infants were two to three times more likely than White infants to have had no well-baby care at all.

Thus the 1989–1990 outbreaks of measles demonstrate that despite the fact that a disease can be prevented almost completely, using economical and safe practices, it won't be prevented unless (1) the public believes that the disease is a serious and direct danger, (2) the barrier of cost is removed, (3) the convenience of obtaining the immunization is real and well known, and (4) there is a tracking system so that both the recipient and provider know the immunization status of the person and the population. Information from other countries indicates that these pre-conditions are best accomplished with a national, voluntary, free (to the immediate consumer) immunization program which is a part of a national, comprehensive, health care program, and which has preventive medicine as its highest priority [9].

After reviewing relevant available data, the National Vaccine Advisory Committee [13] made a number of recommendations addressed to improving the current situation:

1. additional federal financial support should be provided through immunization grants to state and local health departments to enhance the vaccine delivery infrastructure;
2. vigorous efforts should be made, including legislation if necessary, to assure that insurers provide or reimburse for immunizations as a part of their basic health package;
3. Medicaid and its child health component, the early and periodic screen-

ing, detection, and treatment (EPSDT) program, should be integrally involved in tracking children in need of immunizations and providing adequate reimbursement for that service;

4. Medicaid should assess immunization levels of clients served by individual providers as a measure of quality of care and assure compliance with federal EPSDT requirements;

5. state EPSDT programs should comply with federal guidelines and make aggressive efforts to enroll families, recruit and retain health providers, and provide appointment scheduling and transportation assistance as a part of this effort;

6. health departments should reach out to volunteer groups and community organizations to build grass-roots support for adequate resources for immunization and to enhance local requests for and prioritization of immunization.

The National Vaccine Advisory Committee should itself, it reported, issue a formal set of minimum standards for immunization in collaboration with the Interagency Coordinating Group to Improve Access to Immunization and private-sector groups. This Coordinating Group should develop and implement a coordinated plan to assure high immunization levels for those they serve. Federal participation, the committee reported, is needed to support a determination of the immunization status of recipients of aid from the Program for Women, Infants, and Children (WIC) and Aid to Families with Dependent Children, particularly those in urban areas. The committee urged that children with incomplete immunizations be identified and referred for vaccination with appropriate follow-up, or they should be vaccinated at the site where immunization status was recognized as incomplete.

The committee recommended [9] that the National Vaccine Program assure collaboration through the Centers for Disease Control (CDC) of major health provider organizations, including the American Academy of Pediatrics, the American Medical Association, the American Academy of Family Physicians, and other key physician and nursing organizations in order to develop policies among their members to facilitate immunization. It strongly recommended that state and/or local governments that have not yet done so should enact legislation to mandate appropriate immunization prior to enrollment in licensed day-care centers. It urged that national immunization coverage should be assessed annually through the

National Health Interview Survey. Immunization coverage assessments should be required in all states and should be conducted in high-risk urban and rural areas. The CDC, it urged, should explore feasible and economic ways of measuring immunization coverage of 2-year-old children at state and local levels, and federal resources should be used to enhance this surveillance.

The committee also recommended that the two-dose schedule for measles, mumps, and rubella be followed; the first to be given at 15 months and the second on entry to primary, middle, or junior high school. It recommended that a fund be established for outbreak control so that funds would always be immediately available, eliminating the need to wait for emergency appropriations before responding to an outbreak. It pointed out that the two-dose schedule is a long-term solution and its full impact would not be achieved for 7–13 years. Finally, it noted that optimal measles prevention requires greater knowledge about how best to provide vaccine and more information for caregivers about measles virus, measles disease, and the properties of measles vaccine. Therefore, more studies on immunization-program operations and outcomes should be designed to determine the most cost-effective programs of vaccine coverage. Within this recommendation, it noted that laboratory and epidemiologic studies should be conducted to address the problem of measles in highly vaccinated populations and especially in young children. Such studies might include the development of techniques to rapidly diagnose measles and to measure protective immunity. Studies of disease and vaccine strains of measles should be done to ensure that existing vaccines continue to provide a high degree of protection against the naturally occurring measles virus. Studies of the response to the second dose of measles vaccine provided at various ages and intervals are also needed.

The committee concluded by pointing out that the entirety of the recommendations they had made could be funded for $50 million annually, the results of which, as we have seen, would in all probability have a very high benefit-to-cost ratio.

These are important and reasonable, if stopgap, recommendations. Until this country has a comprehensive, coordinated system of health care that establishes preventive medicine as a top priority and funds it adequately, these recommendations should be implemented. We have had our lessons; if we have learned from them and if we act on them, our future can be relieved of the plague of measles.

Editors' Note

Few medical technologies actually show a profit—save more money than they cost—but vaccines for preventing measles do. It is important to understand just how effective the vaccine is. When a susceptible child is exposed to a case of measles, the chance is about 90 percent that the susceptible child will get measles. But when an immunized (vaccinated) child is exposed to a case the chance of getting measles is only about 2–5 percent.

We used to have about 4 million susceptibles a year, and therefore about that many cases of measles. With the introduction of measles vaccine, in just a few years the number of cases per year was brought down to about 7,000. Over a twenty-year period starting in 1963, about 5,000 deaths and 17,000 cases of mental retardation were averted, and a savings of $5 billion from reductions in later health care and increased productivity was realized.

Despite the success of vaccination, measles made a comeback in the United States in 1989 and 1990. Those who got measles were largely children who should have been vaccinated and were not, even though, as reported in this chapter, most had had a chance to be vaccinated. Indeed, on average they had seven chances, none of which were taken. Unless measles is prevented it will generate deaths, mental retardation, and deafness, and it will have especially severe consequences among the poor. The public needs better education in the severity of consequences of measles, and society needs to lower the barriers to preventative measures. Some of these barriers are perceived to be: failure to vaccinate vulnerable children on schedule; lack of a tracking system for our national preventive services; immunizations only by appointment or physician referral; administrative fees; inconvenient clinic hours and location; and language and cultural problems.

A new health care system will need a preventive program as its highest priority: we must track children for their shots and make immunization convenient for all and free to those who cannot otherwise afford them. Special efforts are needed to bring equal participation to minority groups, as has been done for hypertension. When we pass up a chance to make a societal profit through the medical system, we are being nearsighted.

10

Treatment of Hypertension

SIDNEY KLAWANSKY

Introduction

Hypertension is a silent killer. Individuals typically do not experience any symptoms of elevated blood pressure, even while the pressure is damaging arterial walls in the heart, brain, kidneys, and other organs.

Because of the long and silent period preceding manifestation of the disease, it was not until epidemiological studies in the 1960s followed large groups of people over long periods of time that the serious damage caused by hypertension became clear. These studies, including the Framingham Heart Study in Massachusetts [1, 2] and the Tecumseh Study in Michigan [3], heralded the modern period of hypertension detection and treatment. The data in these studies were consistent with the idea that hypertension markedly increases the mortality risk from stroke, kidney failure, coronary artery disease, and congestive heart failure.

Hypertension in individuals may begin relatively early in life, but its symptoms, sometimes including sudden death, usually will not occur until many years later. Because of the wide discrepancy in time of silent onset of the disease and occurrence of lethal events, the detection and treatment of hypertension present special and continuing challenges to medicine.

Stroke is a major consequence of uncontrolled hypertension. About one-third of stroke victims die immediately or soon after onset. A high proportion of the remaining two-thirds suffer debilitating physiological and psychological damage, including inability to walk, slurred speech, and difficulty in forming and expressing ideas. While there is often some improvement in the weeks following stroke, the recovered patient is often subject to dependency and depression.

While the adverse outcomes of uncontrolled hypertension can be catastrophic, hypertension is a condition that can now be treated effectively. The efforts in detection and treatment of hypertension represent a historic, cooperative interplay among individuals in basic science, epidemiology, clinical technology assessment, medical institutions, and government. The change in hypertension from a poorly recognized and grossly inadequately treated disease to a well-recognized and treated disease has occurred over the past twenty or thirty years, during the professional careers of many currently practicing physicians.

In the main, there has been a sound scientific basis for changes in clinical practice that the medical leadership has recommended to practitioners. There has been an impressive evolution of program objectives by a sequence of government-sponsored commissions comprising leading medical experts. These commissions have taken into account new results in basic science, epidemiology, and clinical technology assessment and have helped move these results into routine medical practice. In turn, epidemiological and clinical observations have been fed back to basic science and promoted a sound science policy for directing research into the possible basic mechanisms of hypertension.

Epidemiological evidence suggests that the connection between hypertension and stroke is stronger than that between hypertension and heart attacks. Therefore, tracking the trends in incidence of stroke is probably a reasonable way to assess the impact of improvements in detection and treatment of hypertension. Data from the National Center for Health Statistics and other sources indicate that incidence and mortality from strokes has been declining since the 1970s. While the reduction of other risk factors, such as fat intake and smoking, have undoubtedly helped decrease the stroke rate, more widespread detection and treatment of hypertension has made a major contribution [4].

The Meaning and Prevalence of Hypertension

Hypertension means high blood pressure. Blood pressure is conventionally given as systolic blood pressure over diastolic blood pressure, both in millimeters of mercury (mm Hg). Desirable blood pressure is thought to approximate 120 mm Hg/80 mm Hg, or 120/80. The diastolic blood pressure, the lower number, corresponds to the steady-state pressure in the arterial vascular system. This is the portion of the blood vessels that carries the blood away from the heart to the various organ systems; in other words, the steady diastolic pressure keeps the body's organs bathed in blood. The systolic blood pressure, the higher number, is the pressure generated by the forceful contraction of the left ventricle, the powerful heart chamber that ejects the blood from the heart into the arterial vessel system via the aorta.

Either diastolic blood pressure, systolic blood pressure, or both pressures may be too high. For a long time, a person was defined as having hypertension if systolic blood pressure was equal to or greater than 160 mm Hg, and/or if diastolic blood pressure was equal to or greater than 95 mm Hg, and/or if the person was currently taking antihypertensive medication. However, the precise levels of blood pressure that are considered high have been changing with time. In the recent past, researchers have drawn attention to individuals with borderline hypertension, which includes those having diastolic blood pressure 90–95 mm Hg or systolic blood pressure equal to or greater than 140 mm Hg and less than 160 mm Hg and not taking antihypertensive medication. There is substantial evidence that these individuals can reduce their risk of complications of hypertension if they are treated. (As of January 1994, the categories used for definition are based on diastolic blood pressure; these are mild, 90–104 mm Hg; moderate, 105–114; and severe, 115 and over.)

The second National Health and Nutrition Examination Survey, 1976–1980 (NHANES II) [5], estimated that 25.1 million civilian, noninstitutionalized adults in the United States had hypertension. This number corresponds to an overall prevalence of 17.7 percent. Prevalence increases steadily with age from a low of 2.0 percent for adults ages 18–24 to a high of 45.1 percent for adults ages 65–74 years [5]. Table 10-1 demonstrates that at higher ages, Blacks tend to have a higher prevalence of hypertension than Whites, and that for both Blacks and Whites prevalence rises steadily with age.

The prevalence of hypertension tends to become higher with age in a greater proportion of women than men. Black women in particular experience the most dramatic increase in hypertension, reaching a level of 72.8 per 100 for ages 65–74. Black women of ages 45–64 have roughly twice the prevalence of hypertension of White women of comparable age. Part of this difference may be accounted for by the higher rate of obesity among Black women.

According to NHANES II [5], in addition to the 25.1 million adults aged

Table 10-1. Prevalence rates per 100 for hypertension.

Age group	Whites		Blacks		All groups combined
	Males	Females	Males	Females	
18–24	2.9	0.9	2.4	3.2	2.0
25–34	8.9	3.7	13.3	7.3	6.6
35–44	12.1	8.9	23.8	26.9	12.2
45–54	26.2	21.6	26.0	58.3	25.4
55–64	31.3	34.4	46.4	60.1	34.7
65–74	37.5	48.3	42.9	72.8	45.1
18–74	17.1	16.6	21.1	29.5	17.7

Source: Table 5 in Drizd, Dannenberg, and Engel [5].

18–74 with definite or clear-cut hypertension, there were 17.1 million adults of those ages with borderline hypertension. The overall prevalence of borderline disease was 12.0 percent and, as with definite hypertension, the prevalence increased with age, from 7.0 percent for ages 18–24 to 19.3 percent for ages 65–74. While there is evidence that these individuals can reduce their risk of serious adverse events, such as stroke or heart attack, by drug therapy, the value of medication must be weighed against the potential side effects inherent in long-term therapy.

Treatment

During the early 1960s, only about one in six hypertensives was both aware of being hypertensive and adequately treated for it. Within the hypertensive population, nearly half did not even know that they had hypertension [6]. Since then, the history of scientific, clinical, and educational efforts to understand and treat hypertension stands as a landmark in the history of medicine. The story of the development of drug therapies for hypertension highlights two major goals: (1) the synthesis of specific classes of drugs to deal with each of the proposed major causal mechanisms for hypertension and (2) the concurrent effort to eliminate the side effects associated with each of the classes.

Until the 1950s, hypertension had no safe and effective outpatient treatment. The adverse side effects of the potent antihypertensive agents available before that time militated against their routine use. In the late 1950s, diuretics (drugs that cause the kidney to excrete more fluid) came into use as the first effective antihypertensive agents with an acceptably low level of adverse side effects.

In the late 1960s, at the time that epidemiological studies were documenting the devastating effect of untreated hypertension, the Veterans Administration Cooperative Study on Antihypertensive Agents conducted a large randomized, double-blind, placebo-controlled trial on the efficacy of therapy in reducing mortality and morbidity [7–9]. Those treated with placebo were followed for 15.7 months, and the drug-treated group was followed for 20.7 months. For the 143 patients at high risk with diastolic blood pressure (DBP) 115–129 mm Hg, the drug used for active treatment was hydrochlorothiazide plus reserpine plus hydralazine hydrochloride. Mean diastolic blood pressure in the treated group of 73 fell 28.1 mm Hg, from 121.2 mm Hg to 93.1 mm Hg. The mean diastolic blood pressure in the control group of 70 fell 2.5 mm Hg.

There were more than ten times as many severe morbid or mortal events in the placebo-treated or control group than in the drug-treated group (27 vs. 2). There were four deaths in the control group but none in the treated group. Serious vascular events caused damage to patients' eyes, brains, and hearts.

In the large clinical trial studying hypertensives in the moderately ele-

---

An Uncommon Side Effect?

Like most human endeavors, research has its lighter side, too. We are pleased to report here an unusual experience concerning the effect of reserpine on animal behavior.

After reading in a pet journal that reserpine produced striking colors in angelfish, one of the editors of this volume put a tiny dose in a tank containing two angelfish. Angelfish are rather aggressive, and the larger one of the pair had always bullied the smaller. In this instance, too, the larger one prevailed and got most of the reserpine. Both fish soon acquired beautiful dark colors, but the big bully no longer charged after the smaller fish. For several weeks the bullying was reversed, and the small fish successfully chased the big one. Eventually, though, the colors faded, and thereafter the big fish resumed its place at the top of the pecking order.

vated range (DBP 90–114 mm Hg), severe events occurred in 18 percent of the control group but in only 5 percent of the drug-treated group [8]. More than twice as many deaths occurred in the control group as in the treated group. Treatment was more effective in preventing the complications of congestive heart failure and stroke than in preventing the complications of coronary artery disease. Those with higher initial blood pressure appeared to benefit more from treatment than those in the lower part of the range before the study began. The V.A. Cooperative Study established that treatment can systematically lower dangerously high blood pressure and clearly demonstrated the lifesaving effect of lowering elevated blood pressure.

In 1971, the National Institutes of Health embarked on the High Blood Pressure Education Program. By 1974, after the program had been in effect for only two or three years, the proportion of patients who did not know that they were hypertensive dropped by about half, and there was a 50 percent increase in the number of hypertensives who were adequately treated. Particularly in the Black community, where identification of and treatment of hypertension was taken as a particular challenge in light of the high prevalence, there was a tremendous improvement in the diagnosis and treatment of hypertension. There was a decline in the incidence of heart disease and especially of stroke.

In 1975, the Joint Committee on the Detection, Evaluation and Treatment of High Blood Pressure (JNC I) issued one of the first guidelines for treatment: treat all adults with diastolic blood pressure (DBP) equal to or greater than 105 mm Hg and those with DBP 90–104 mm Hg in combination with other risk factors, such as diabetes [10].

In 1979, the Hypertension Detection and Follow-Up Program (HDFP) published its results [11, 12]. This trial compared the effects of a systematic treatment program (Stepped Care) and referral to community-based medical care (Referred Care). Stepped Care means that the physician prescribes an initial or first-line drug and then steps up to the addition of a back-up or second-line drug, if needed for blood pressure control. Referred Care means referral to the patient's regular doctor with no special instructions.

Those persons with diastolic blood pressure of 90 mm Hg or more assigned to Stepped Care achieved consistently better control of their hypertension. This group showed a 17 percent reduction in overall mortality, a 45 percent reduction in deaths from stroke, and a 26 percent reduction in deaths from heart attack, as compared with those in the Referred Care group. Mortality was also considerably lower for the Stepped

Care subgroup with mild hypertension (DBP 90–104 mm Hg) compared with the corresponding Referred Care group.

In 1980, following a review of the results of the HDFP, the JNC II report was issued. This report recommended treatment of persons with diastolic blood pressure of 90 mm Hg or more (borderline hypertension) and updated the Stepped Care treatment guidelines to include the beta-blocker class of drugs. These new guidelines also recommended that obese patients reduce their weight and that hypertensive patients, in general, reduce their salt intake as part of the total management of hypertension. (As new information is acquired, the Joint National Committee continues to revise the recommendations.)

Classes of Antihypertensive Drugs and JNC Recommendations

With traditional antihypertensive therapy, part of the trade-off of medication was that a reduction of blood pressure was sometimes bought at the price of a small but significant increase in fatty substances in the blood. In addition, some antihypertensive drugs may also have been ineffective in reducing the enlargement of the heart induced by hypertension.

Investigators have dedicated a very active research effort to the development of new families of antihypertensive drugs. Especially prominent among these families are the beta-blockers, the calcium channel blockers, and the angiotensin converting enzyme (ACE) inhibitors. These drugs, notably the ACE inhibitors and to a lesser degree the calcium channel blockers, appear to cause a reduction of heart enlargement and, one hopes, will reduce long-term hypertension mortality.

Calcium channel blockers are so named because they interfere with the passage of calcium ions through the membranes of the cells in the heart wall. This movement of ions is part of the physiological process of heart muscle contraction. Interfering with this process has the effect of reducing the force of contraction of the heart. In a similar manner, these drugs also affect the tension in the walls of the arterial blood vessels, reducing the vascular constriction and thereby reducing elevated blood pressure.

Among the new classes of drugs, however, the most promising may well be the ACE inhibitors. These agents inhibit the formation, from a blood protein normally present, of angiotensin II, a substance that exerts a powerful constricting force on the arterial blood vessels. This constriction of the arterial blood vessels raises blood pressure. Studies have shown that ACE inhibitors are effective in lowering blood pressure and treating heart failure. As a class these drugs have relatively few side effects. They do not induce adverse metabolic changes, such as increasing blood sugar or fat content, that could negate the beneficial effects of reducing blood pressure. The generally few side effects means that ACE inhibitors improve the quality of life for persons on antihypertensive medication. It is generally agreed that physicians should treat hypertension in the elderly. Because they have few side effects, ACE inhibitors are thought to be good agents for treating elderly hypertensives.

Therapy with ACE inhibitors alone often may not be completely effective in reducing blood pressure in hypertensive patients. Controlled studies have shown that combining ACE inhibitors with low doses of diuretics can provide effective blood pressure reduction in the great majority of patients while avoiding the undesirable side effects associated with diuretics.

The report of the JNC III was published in 1984. This report, reflecting changes in objectives and target populations, emphasized the importance of directing screening programs primarily at high-risk groups. JNC III recommended the increased use of behavioral and dietary methods, such as salt reduction and weight control, as early treatment measures as well as during long-term management of hypertension. The Stepped Care recommendations were updated to include the beta-blockers as Step 1 agents and the calcium channel blockers and ACE inhibitors as appropriate agents for later steps.

Effectiveness of Treatments for Known Hypertensives

To assess the effectiveness of reaching and treating individuals diagnosed with hypertension, we can take advantage of two cross-sectional surveys conducted during the period 1971–1980. The first survey was the first National Health and Nutrition Examination Survey (NHANES I) conducted over 1971–1974. The second survey, NHANES II, was conducted over 1976–1980. Because the methodologies of the two surveys were similar, we can make comparisons across the time period 1971–1980 spanned by them.

Figure 10-1 displays the percentages of males and females with hypertension who were treated, by age and race. Note that although Blacks are burdened with a high prevalence of hypertension (Table 10-1), medicine has identified and treated a higher percentage of hypertensive Blacks than Whites for both sexes and for both younger and older age groups. At the time of NHANES II (1976–1980), for both males and females, a higher proportion of hypertensive Blacks than Whites were receiving medications.

In spite of improvements in identifying and treating hypertensives in

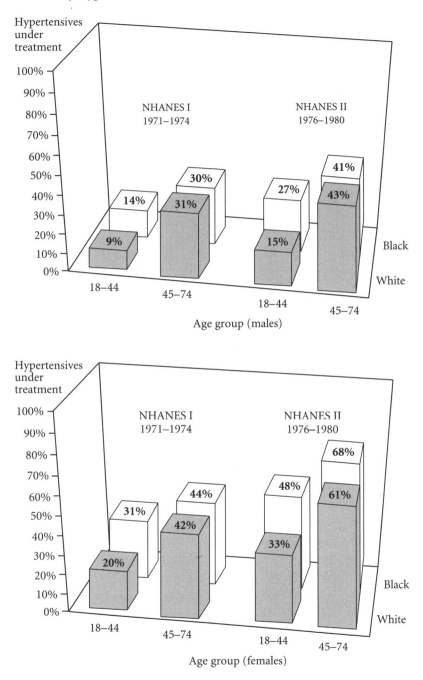

Figure 10-1. A comparison of percentage of hypertensives under treatment in the NHANES I study (1971–1974) and the NHANES II study (1976–1980) by race, sex, and age. (Data from the National Health and Nutrition Examination Survey, or NHANES, as reported by Drizd, Dannenberg, and Engel [5].)

the period of 1976–1980 as compared with 1971–1974, however, the overall pattern of low proportions of young hypertensives under treatment has persisted. Only 9 percent of White and 14 percent of Black hypertensive males in the age range 18–44 were under treatment in the period 1971–1974, rising to 15 percent and 27 percent respectively by 1976–1980.

Trends in Cardiovascular Deaths

In 1968, 54 percent of all deaths in the United States were due to cardiovascular disease; 35 percent of all deaths were from coronary heart disease and 11 percent were from strokes. By 1982, only 49 percent, or less than half, of all deaths were due to cardiovascular disease, with 28 percent being due to coronary heart disease and 8 percent to stroke [13].

The decline in deaths from stroke by the 1980s was dramatic; it was apparent among White men and women and among Black men and women. Black men aged 55–64 still have about three times the stroke rate of White men of comparable age, however, and Black women aged 55–64 have almost three times the rate of White women. For all groups combined, however, the death rate from stroke for ages 55–64 is only about one-third of what it was in the 1950s. A major contribution to this reduction has been the widespread detection and treatment of hypertension.

Common fatal events associated with hypertension are strokes, heart attacks, and congestive heart failure. In addition to hypertension, smoking, elevated cholesterol levels, and lack of exercise may increase the risk of heart attacks and strokes. The reduction of each of these risk factors contributes to the observed lowering in the death rate from cardiovascular disease. The cardiovascular event that is probably most closely connected with hypertension is stroke. The observed downward trend in stroke rates over the past 20–30 years is probably an important result of the increased rate of detection and treatment of hypertension. A recent meta-analysis by the Oxford epidemiology group [14] found that there was no lower threshold for the benefit of lowering the stroke rate by reducing blood pressure. Reduction of blood pressure, even where initial pressure is normal, produces the benefit of a reduction in the rate of stroke.

Costs of Ambulatory Hypertension Treatment

Assuming that 15 million Americans are under treatment at a cost of $500 per patient year, aggregate costs of treating hypertension in ambulatory patients are estimated to be about $7.5 billion per year [15]. The cost of

$500 per person covers office visits, medications, and laboratory costs. A study of costs of hypertension clinics in the Veterans Administration system found that the cost of ambulatory care was about $325 per patient year in a 1984 study [16]. Forty-nine percent of costs were for office visits, 30 percent for medications, and 15 percent for laboratory examinations. Note that medication costs in the V.A. system are far below those in other sectors because the V.A. is a bulk purchaser of pharmaceuticals.

Depending on the agents prescribed, the costs per year of medication vary dramatically, from about $15 per year for generic diuretics and $240 for newer beta-blockers to $410 for ACE inhibitors and $560 for calcium channel blockers, as demonstrated by a 1989 study [15]. There is evidence that because of the more benign side effects, physicians are more commonly prescribing the newer and more expensive ACE inhibitors and calcium channel blockers, frequently substituting them for the traditional diuretics or beta-blockers. The cost-effectiveness perspective suggests that the newer drugs, because of their much higher costs, are best suited for patients who are not adequately controlled on less expensive agents and for patients who cannot tolerate the latter's side effects. If this perspective were shared by all, physicians would not initiate therapy with the new, expensive agents unless these conditions are met.

In light of the wide variation in the cost of treatment, the cost-effectiveness perspective is consistent with initiating pharmacological therapy by prescribing one of the low-cost diuretics, which, with office and laboratory costs, would be about $108–128 per year, or a beta-blocker, with a total cost of $201–262 per year. Physicians would substitute higher-cost agents, such as ACE inhibitors at a cost of about $378 per year, only if the cheaper drugs didn't work or caused unwanted side effects. Note that the difference of about $270 per patient year between the lowest- and the highest-cost pharmaceutical therapies amounts to about a quarter of a billion dollars for each million hypertensive patients treated [15].

Weinstein and Stason [17] examined the cost-effectiveness of treating known hypertensive individuals with special attention to the age and sex of the patient, the pre-treatment level of diastolic hypertension, and the degree of adherence to the long-term medical regimen. The study reported three major conclusions [15]. The first is that hypertension treatment does not pay for itself in savings in terms of the medical cost of strokes or heart attacks prevented. Treatment appears to recover only about 27 percent of the cost of treating moderate hypertension (diastolic blood pressure equal to or greater than 105 mm Hg) and only 15 percent of the costs of treating mild hypertension (diastolic blood pressure of 90–104 mm Hg). The value of treating hypertension must be measured in terms of the human lives saved and disability avoided.

Second, the cost-effectiveness of treatment is directly related to the pre-treatment level of diastolic blood pressure. Cost-effectiveness is measured in dollar costs of antihypertensive drugs minus the savings from strokes and other morbid events that have been prevented. Cost-effectiveness for treatment of cardiovascular diseases like hypertension typically is in the range of tens of thousands of dollars per Quality Adjusted Life Year (QALY). The measurement of a QALY takes into account the idea that an increased year of life for a hypertensive patient with medication side effects or disability as a result of stroke is worth less than a year of full health.

The cost of treating hypertension is of the order of $500 dollars per year. By comparison, the amount of money needed to purchase a volume of care that will yield an additional year of life for a hypertensive person will be a much higher number. This higher amount includes the discounted sum of the annual amounts of care for all the years on treatment.

Weinstein and Stason calculated that in 1984 dollars, full adherence to medical regimens cost $45,000, $22,000 and $9,000 per QALY for pre-treatment diastolic blood pressures of 90–94, 95–104, and 105 or higher, respectively. These calculations suggest that treatment of individuals with diastolic blood pressure greater than 105 mm Hg is more than twice as cost-effective as is treatment of those with diastolic blood pressure 90–104 mm Hg. Not everyone finds the QALY approach acceptable, but we will not pursue this issue further here except to say that persons with such a disease may regard the approach as one that almost always underestimates the value of treatment to them.

Third, cost-effectiveness ratios are roughly one-third higher in dollars per QALY when expected failure to adhere to medical regimens or breaks in continuity of care are factored into the calculations.

To put these cost-effectiveness ratios in perspective, Weinstein and Stason note that the treatment of mild hypertension (90–104 mm Hg) is about as effective as coronary artery bypass graft surgery (CABG) in patients with disease in two separate, major coronary arteries and who are unresponsive to medical therapy.

Another use for cost-effectiveness analysis is to help allocate resources among the various steps between the undiagnosed, asymptomatic hypertensive and the adequately treated patient. For example, because the prevalence of hypertension increases with age, it is therefore less expensive to find the same number of hypertensive individuals among the elderly [18]. It follows that as a group of undiagnosed individuals ages, more resources can be shifted from screening to treatment for the same or increased level of societal benefit.

Comparison of Policy Recommendations and Survey Data

The comparison of survey data with the recommendations of cost-effectiveness analysis of treatment of hypertension suggests that the health care system has closed gaps regarding treatment by race and needs to focus on the issue of treating two groups that are relatively underserved: men and young people. Because side effects of currently available antihypertensive drugs may reduce compliance with treatment programs, the advent of new drugs with even milder side effects may close the treatment gap with respect to younger men.

Improving the Cost-effectiveness of Hypertension Treatment

Identifying individuals as hypertensives should not rely on a single elevated reading. A Gallup survey indicated that as many as 43 percent of physicians in the United States who treated hypertension started drug therapy because of a diastolic blood pressure measurement of 90–99 on a single office visit [19]. According to the Joint National Council report of 1985, at least one-third of such patients will not have sustained hypertension. A related issue involves "white-coat hypertension." In one study, 20 percent of patients with persistently elevated clinical pressures, as measured by their physicians using a standard sphygmomanometer, did not meet the criteria for hypertension during automatic, ambulatory 24-hour blood pressure monitoring. Clearly, we need to be very careful in establishing a diagnosis of hypertension.

The Gallup poll revealed that for about 14 percent of patients, cost was the most important factor in their consideration of antihypertensive medications and that problems in paying for medications (25 percent) were even more important than side effects (14 percent). In the survey, only 59 percent of patients had insurance policies that covered medications. For patients whose incomes were below $15,000, this figure fell to 44 percent [20]. Since cost of medication is an important consideration for some hypertensive patients, it seems cost-effective to provide lower-cost medication where possible, if it can provide good blood pressure control with acceptably small side effects. For patients in the diastolic blood pressure range of 90–99 mm Hg, the trade-offs between the benefits and risks of treatment become less clear-cut. Loss of libido in the case of beta-blockers and the tendency of diuretic agents to increase serum cholesterol need to be considered in the risk-benefit calculation.

This cost-effectiveness perspective strongly suggests that physicians should encourage the initiation of nonpharmacological treatments, including salt restriction, exercise, and weight reduction, before embarking on drug therapy. If a patient's lipoprotein values remain high, it may be appropriate to consider pharmacological intervention to adjust these values as well as to lower blood pressure. Because of the multiple risk factors affecting coronary artery disease (CAD), it is important to look upon the treatment of hypertension as a measure that needs to be coordinated with the treatment of other major coronary risk factors.

Improvement in Life Expectancy from Detection and Treatment of Hypertension

In an overview of 420,000 individuals in nine major prospective observational studies [14], the Oxford epidemiology research group found that, on average, a usual diastolic blood pressure that was lower by 5–6 mm Hg was associated with about 35–40 percent fewer strokes and 20–25 percent less coronary artery disease. There was no evidence of any "threshold" below which lower levels of blood pressure were not associated with lower risks of stroke and CAD.

A parallel overview analyzed 14 randomized control trials of antihypertensive therapy with a mean treatment duration of 5 years [21]. Diastolic blood pressure groupings for subjects upon entry to the trials ranged from elevated but less than 110 mm Hg to elevated and greater than 115 mm Hg. A reduction in diastolic blood pressure of 5–6 mm Hg due to the therapy reduced strokes by 42 percent within a window of about 2–3 years, suggesting that the stroke reduction from treatment is achieved rapidly.

The National Center for Health Statistics published a set of life tables for 1979–1981 that calculated the expected gain in life expectancy due to the elimination of specified causes of death for those who would have died of the disease [22]. Table E of that report estimates that elimination of hypertension would produce a gain of 10 years in life expectancy at birth.

By way of comparison, the table indicates that elimination of diabetes would provide a gain of 12 years in life expectancy.

These estimates of lives saved reflect the dramatic improvements that medical research and practice have produced over the past 20–30 years in the detection and treatment of hypertension. The achievements to date provide a solid base from which to continue focused efforts to eliminate the remaining preventable morbidity and mortality from hypertension.

Editors' Note

By describing the evolution of the treatment of hypertension since its initial recognition as a treatable disease, this chapter illustrates the iterative, lengthy, and complex developments required to reap health benefits for patients who perceive no adverse symptoms of their "disease." Some diseases can be regarded as essentially present or absent, but hypertension seems now to be present in nearly everyone, in the sense that reduced blood pressure seems to be almost universally beneficial. Thus the definition of who is diseased (or ought to be treated) depends on the trade-off between nuisance, costs, and side effects of treatment with the increase in life expectancy and improvement in long-run quality of life to be gained by treatment.

Nearly 60 million people in the United States would benefit from treatment for hypertension, reducing their incidence of damage to blood vessels, heart, and brain and gaining perhaps ten years in life expectancy. Through remarkable sustained cooperation among health researchers, basic scientists, medical practitioners, patients, the pharmaceutical industry, insurance companies, and governmental health agencies, great improvements in care have been achieved over the past two decades. In addition to new drugs and treatments, there have been improvements in casefinding and dissemination of information about managing hypertension, especially in minority communities.

Unusually diverse sources of information have contributed to this campaign. Disease registries, epidemiologic studies, and sample surveys have identified groups especially at risk and suggested groups for whom treatment might be effective, while randomized, controlled trials have verified that specific blood pressure groups do benefit from the treatments.

A recurring problem in health care stems from the availability of a pair of effective treatments such that one is much more expensive and somewhat more effective than the other. Although the problem of deciding which treatment to choose in such a dilemma comes up frequently, society does not yet seem to have grasped this nettle. Yet it should if it is to have an affordable and effective universal health care system.

Reaping the benefits of successful treatments for a silent disease requires a complex, multifactorial program, one that can identify appropriate groups for treatment, educate them, and maintain their therapies. The fact that the hypertension educational program has been more effective for minorities than for the general population deserves attention, because we need to find out how to adapt its successful methods to programs directed against other diseases. Since, as always, young patients (aged 18–44) are difficult to recruit into medical studies, we must also learn how to educate them about the risk of hypertension.

This chapter brings out several points about the kind of broad, multifactorial programs needed to overcome diseases like hypertension. For example, frequent changes in guidelines for therapy based on new evidence must not undermine the credibility of the treatment program; rather, they must be seen as the natural result of advances in medical knowledge. The high cost of effective drugs, which creates a barrier to access, is a problem in the treatment of many diseases, and the search for less expensive and nearly as effective drugs for a variety of diseases needs more attention.

This chapter also provides an illustration of productive, long-term cooperative programs among basic scientists, health workers, industry, and government. Furthermore, it highlights the need for technology assessment—finding out which groups are benefited by treatment and to what degree, as well as which drugs are effective and to what degree—even for what may be considered routine care.

After about forty years of development, the program for managing hypertension offers a potential increase of ten years in life expectancy to those most afflicted with the disease, who make up a substantial portion of the whole population. It should therefore serve as a model of a successful attempt to monitor and deliver health care.

PART F

The Delivery of Routine Care: Visual and Dental Health

We have emphasized in this book the need for rigorous evaluation of medical innovations to determine whether they merit wide distribution. Because our resources are limited, the delivery of routine care must also be managed wisely. Decisions about the allocation of services depend not only on an assessment of their efficacy but also on the prevalence of specific diseases or conditions. In the two cases discussed in this section—weakening eyesight and dental decay—the monitoring of health status is essential to the delivery of achievable benefits.

Natural changes in the eye over time, plus imperfections present at birth, produce near- or farsightedness or astigmatism in nearly every sighted person who reaches adulthood. Inexpensive lenses can be readily fitted to improve visual acuity, thus improving quality of life. Nearly everyone benefits from lenses at some time in life, and half of those using them wear them all the time. Few medical aids are as widely used as lenses, yet few health insurance programs cover the cost of detection and correction of eye problems. For the case of eye care, technology assessment is required less to evaluate the treatment than to find the best, most cost-effective way to deliver a proven treatment.

Dental care is also an example of a treatment whose worth has been proven. Substantial changes in dental theory and practice have reduced the rates of decay and loss of teeth with successive generations. The effects of prevention have been most successful. New materials, the use of analgesics, and payment through insurance have made dental care more widespread and less feared. The numbers of people who have lost all their teeth have decreased drastically, as has the number using dentures. At the same time, more teeth survive to be worn out, and so we have the paradox that improved dental health may lead to a greater need for repair and restoration of teeth. Maintaining effective delivery of the broad spectrum of dental services is the challenge for the future of dentistry, and continual evaluation of the delivery of care will be needed to meet that challenge.

11

The Contributions of Lenses to Visual Health

GEORGIANNA MARKS, FREDERICK MOSTELLER,
MARIE-A McPHERSON, AND GRACE WYSHAK

Background

Among the many benefits that medical innovations have conferred upon mankind, few have contributed so broadly and yet so substantially as eyeglasses and contact lenses. Correction of errors in vision has meant the difference for many people between isolation or dependency on others and active membership in society. Yet the subtle contributions of glasses to a person's quality of life are often undocumented, because they lack the lifesaving drama of some drugs and medical interventions. Even plain safety glasses prevent disabling injuries and make certain hazardous occupations possible. Glasses and contact lenses are now medical benefits taken for granted, but imagine the consequences of a world without them. Millions could not read or drive a car, work with computers, or safely perform many occupational tasks. As medical interventions go, lenses and their fitting are comparatively inexpensive to provide, though priceless to the person who uses them.

Lenses correct a variety of visual problems, and in this chapter we primarily discuss four of the most common: nearsightedness (myopia), farsightedness (including hyperopia and presbyopia), and astigmatism. Myopia is one of the major causes of visual disability. Until the development and wide availability of glasses and contact lenses, the myopic person's only remedy for clear distance vision was squinting. Farsightedness in older persons, presbyopia, is caused by a stiffness in the human lens, whereas farsightedness in younger persons, hyperopia, is not due to stiffness but to an inability of the lens for other reasons to accommodate sufficiently to focus the image at the retina. Astigmatism results from irregular shapes of corneas and produces blurred vision.

All four major refractive errors—nearsightedness, farsightedness in young people, astigmatism, and presbyopia—can be corrected by lenses. Nearsightedness is improved by concave lenses, farsightedness by convex lenses, astigmatism by cylindrical lenses, and presbyopia by bifocals. For people who have to adjust their eyesight to several distances, trifocals are becoming more common.

This chapter documents the magnitude of these vision problems in modern society and the extent of amelioration that lenses offer, including discussion of the relation of near and distance vision to quality of life. Nearly all who pass the age of 45 years in the United States of America have worn lenses for some purposes at some time in their lives, and among those wearing glasses 53 percent wear them nearly all the time [1].

It is difficult to pinpoint exactly when eyeglasses first appeared. Folklore is rich in anecdotal reports. For the period before the thirteenth century, undocumented theories about the origins and availability of glasses abound. Nevertheless, numerous artifacts, many from China, prove that forms of glasses were available in these earlier periods. For a historical perspective on the origins of glasses, we have relied heavily on the works of James Gregg [2], Bausch & Lomb [3], Lael Tucker Wertenbaker [4], and Brian Curtin [5].

In 1623, Benito Daza de Valdes, a notary of the Inquisition in Seville, Spain, produced an illustrated scientific work on spectacles entitled *Use of Spectacles for All Kinds of Sight*. This work is especially revealing of the knowledge available at the time, because it provides tables assigning lens strength for presbyopes at various ages for both men and women. Gregg [2, p. 22] points to a puzzle: it is difficult to find claimants taking credit for the invention of glasses, whereas most important inventions have many. He suggests the possibility that when glasses first came into use in Europe in the Middle Ages, they may have been seen as a form of magic, and anyone claiming to have invented them would have been persecuted by the established church.

The invention of printing in 1440, followed by a rise in literacy, is believed to have created the need for visual aids in an increasing number of people and to have been the driving force behind the production of glasses. As noted in one history of the industry, "Conditions previous to the Eighteenth Century rendered the use of glasses unnecessary to the majority of individuals. The ability to read and write was a possession of the learned few, and the costliness of glasses made them prohibitive to the average individual" [3].

The Loss of Visual Acuity

Figure 11-1 illustrates how rays of light are processed in the eye. In a normal eye, light entering the eye is focused on the retina and vision is acute, clear. In the myopic eye, the parallel rays of light entering the eye at rest are refracted in such a way as to focus in front of the retina instead of on it. As a consequence, the myopic person cannot perceive distant objects clearly. In 1976 the National Eye Institute found myopia to be the fifth most frequent cause of severe visual impairment and the seventh most frequent cause of legal blindness. Hyperopia is also caused by an error in the refraction of light rays, one that places the focus of the light rays *behind* the retina.

Ophthalmologists classify myopia as physiologic or pathologic. In physiologic myopia (developmental, maturational, or simple school myopia), nearsightedness results from a chance combination of normal refraction components in the eye, such as an increase in curvature of the surfaces of the cornea or lens or an increased axial diameter of the eye attained by normal growth. The blurring of the retinal image in this case is related to the degree of myopia. In pathologic myopia (degenerative, progressive, or malignant myopia), an abnormal development or other aberration of growth interferes with the focusing of light on the retina.

Theories about the etiology of myopia are many. In a review of the possible causes of the condition, Curtin [5] reports that certain factors have a well-established association with the development and prevalence of myopia: heredity, premature birth, malnutrition, acquired systemic disease, and glaucoma. Curtin also reports that the lack of agreement in the literature about the etiology of myopia is mostly due to differences over methodology and choice of the population to be sampled. Because the prevalence of myopia varies naturally with age, he argues, it is inappropriate to compare, for example, the frequency of myopia in a teenage population with that in a middle-aged group.

In a study of visual acuity as it relates to the aging process, Pitts [7] indicates that acuity follows a distinctive pattern of development. From near blindness at birth, an infant acquires a much improved level of acuity

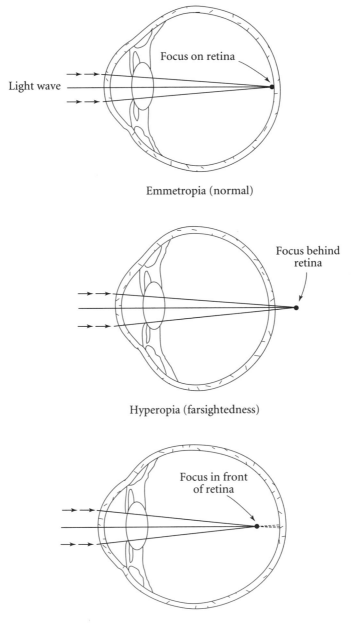

Figure 11-1. The path of light in the normal, myopic, and hyperopic eye. (Adapted from *Vision Research, a National Plan 1983–1987,* from the U.S. Department of Health and Human Services.)

by the first year of life. Gradual improvement occurs from 5 years of age up to sometime between 20–30 years of age, and then acuity remains constant until about 55 years of age, followed by steady decline.

The pathologic causes of the loss in visual acuity seen in later life are related to the aging process and include cataract, macular degeneration, diabetic retinopathy (see Chapter 4), and glaucoma. In this chapter we do not deal with these diseases.

Surveys of Visual Acuity

Researchers of vision face the choice of a standard. Should we ask how well people can see things that are 100 feet away, or 20 feet away, or a few inches? The decision can make a huge difference in how we define blindness. The standard of measure may even lead us to make poor choices in the intent of therapy, as happens when instead of trying to make the most of the vision the patient has we try to meet a hopeless standard. For example, we may need to give someone a small telescope instead of heavier glasses. Nevertheless, for much work in vision two distances have been widely used for assessments: "far," or about 20 feet (or 6 meters), and "near," or about 14 inches, a distance often associated approximately with reading or close work.

The standard of 20 feet is rather practical, because what can be done for vision at that distance matches well with what can be done at longer distances. As a crude rule, 20 feet is an infinite distance in optical theory.

Most readers are familiar with some version of the Snellen chart and with the numerical "score" one receives when asked to read it. A score of 20/20 is associated with "good" vision; 20/40 is associated with poorer but generally adequate vision; and 20/200, very poor vision. The numerator refers to the 20 feet standard distance to a "far" object, and the denominator is the distance people with good vision would have to stand to see equally well what the person tested sees at 20 feet.

The general idea is to rate the vision of subjects by having them read lines of letters of essentially the same size. Near the bottom of the chart is a line corresponding to 20/20, meaning that people who can accurately read this line but not a smaller (lower) line from a distance of 20 feet have "good" vision according to the standard chosen. We will arbitrarily call 20/20 (or 6/6 in metric units) good vision for this exposition. People with better vision may be able to read smaller lines and would get a better score—perhaps 20/15, implying roughly that they can see at 20 feet what

Table 11-1. Mean acuities for far vision (numerator 20 feet) for 577 men in Baltimore Longitudinal Study of Aging, both Presenting and Uncorrected measurements expressed as a Snellen decimal. Respondents wore their own distant-vision glasses for the Presenting measurement and no glasses for the Uncorrected measurement.

Cohort (average age)	Snellen decimal		Difference	Ratio[a]	Percent of sample wearing lenses
	Presenting	Uncorrected			
1895/78.4	0.76	0.51	0.25	1.5	94
1900/74.5	0.85	0.55	0.30	1.5	96
1905/69.5	0.97	0.57	0.40	1.7	98
1910/65.0	1.03	0.62	0.41	1.7	100
1915/60.4	1.04	0.61	0.43	1.7	100
1920/55.9	1.07	0.75	0.32	1.4	98
1925/50.7	1.13	0.70	0.43	1.6	99
1930/46.4	1.15	0.81	0.34	1.4	98
1935/41.7	1.18	0.82	0.36	1.4	88
1940/37.0	1.15	0.74	0.41	1.6	73
1945/33.7	1.18	0.80	0.38	1.5	66

a. Presenting fraction divided by Uncorrected fraction.

Source: Reprinted from N. S. Gittings and J. L. Fozard, "Age related changes in visual acuity," *Experimental Gerontology* 21 (1986), 423–433, copyright 1986, with permission from Pergamon Press Ltd, Headington Hill Hall, Oxford OX3 OBW, UK.

a person with "good" vision would see accurately from 15 feet. Most of our attention is on people who see less well than "good."

If we express the ratio as a decimal, 20/20 corresponds to 1, 20/15 to 1.33, and 20/25 to 0.8. Ratios larger than 1 imply especially acute vision— "hawkeyes"—and ratios less than 1 give some notion of the reduction of visual acuity from the 20/20 standard.

Toward the zero end of the scale, investigators take an interest in just what the person can detect in the way of light and shadow. At this point, when dealing with people having very poor vision, the Snellen approach loses its utility. Although it is tempting and convenient to speak as if a person with a ratio of 0.5 has half the visual acuity of a person with a ratio of 1.0, that probably is an oversimplification.

In the early 1980s, the Baltimore Longitudinal Study of Aging (see Table 11-1) measured visual acuity using the Snellen fractions for people in various birth cohorts. The cohorts grouped births in five-year intervals. The people in the 1895 cohort were born in the years 1895 through 1899. The population sampled was "an upper-middle-class segment of the general population" [8, p. 425]. The researchers tested each person's eyes separately and then reported the acuity for the better eye. They recorded the results under two conditions: "uncorrected" and "presenting." "Presenting" means that the measurement was made with the subjects wearing their own glasses if glasses were used for far vision, and "uncorrected" means that no lenses were worn.

The investigation ran over a period of several years, and most subjects were measured seven times. The report is based on 577 men, though women were added late in the study. Except in the very elderly, men and women turn out to have similar acuities. For all but the oldest three cohorts, the Presenting acuity averaged better than 1, indicating better visual acuity than the standard of 20/20. In the eight oldest cohorts—by 45 years of age—almost everyone wore glasses at their last visit.

Generally speaking, older people had poorer acuity both Presenting and Uncorrected. But the average gain due to glasses was about 0.37, a numerical improvement of over a third. When the Presenting Snellen decimal is near 1, a difference of a third means an improvement of about 10 feet (from what good viewers can see at 30 feet to what they can see at 20 feet) for the average individual. The magnitudes are quite impressive and are reinforced by the percentages of people involved. Except for the oldest two age groups, the improvement from Uncorrected to Presenting is rather consistently in the neighborhood of 0.4, allowing for sampling fluctuations in the groups. Thus the glasses provide a very impressive and consistent gain for distance viewing.

For near viewing, the investigators used a similar sort of Snellen approach but with 14 inches as the standard distance. They found Snellen ratios such as 14/140, 14/70, 14/49, 14/35, . . . 14/17.5, 14/14, 14/10.5 for near vision. Persons with scores worse than 14/140 were assigned scores of 14/280.

Table 11-2 shows the near-viewing comparison with and without glasses. The differences range much more widely for the near condition than for far. Especially in the older groups, the average gains are huge. The test of far vision is carried out at approximately 20 feet (or some optically equivalent distance and size). Near vision is usually measured at 14 inches, but tests usually allow the subjects to set the near work, usually reading,

Table 11-2. Average decimal acuities for near vision (numerator 14 inches), both Presenting and Uncorrected measurements for 11 five-year cohorts. Respondents wore their own near-vision glasses for the Presenting measurement and no glasses for the Uncorrected measurement.

Cohort (average age)	Snellen decimal		Difference	Ratio[a]
	Presenting	Uncorrected		
1895/78.4	0.81	0.35	0.46	2.3
1900/74.5	0.90	0.34	0.56	2.6
1905/69.5	1.02	0.32	0.70	3.2
1910/65.0	1.07	0.40	0.77	2.7
1915/60.4	1.10	0.42	0.68	2.6
1920/55.9	1.12	0.55	0.57	2.0
1925/50.7	1.17	0.66	0.51	1.8
1930/46.4	1.22	0.75	0.57	1.6
1935/41.7	1.24	1.03	0.21	1.2
1940/37.0	1.26	1.06	0.20	1.2
1945/33.7	1.33	1.14	0.19	1.2

a. Presenting fraction divided by the Uncorrected fraction.
Source: Reprinted from N. S. Gittings and J. L. Fozard, "Age related changes in visual acuity," *Experimental Gerontology* 21 (1986), 423–433, copyright 1986, with permission from Pergamon Press Ltd, Headington Hill Hall, Oxford OX3 OBW, UK.

at a distance effective for themselves. As a result, the percentage variation of measures of near vision may be quite substantial.

Discussion given in the National Health Survey on vision in persons 4–74 years [1] tells us that one's visual acuity is largely determined by the performance in the better eye; and many reports give information for the better eye. Table 11-3 gives for various age groups the percent of people whose corrected better eye is 20/20 or better. When people with their usual corrective lenses did not achieve 20/40, the examiner in the National Health Survey gave additional correction where possible. (Among respondents who wore lenses, 90 percent used them for reading, and 62 percent for distance.) The table suggests that males and females have similar patterns of performance at various ages. We should note that these data come from the early 1970s and may not match a current national sample.

Pitts [7] suggests that two factors will assist in maintaining visual acuity

Table 11-3. Percent of population, by age and sex, whose vision is 20/20 or better in the corrected better eye.

Age groups	Men	Women
65–74	32.4	33.3
55–64	58.5	57.4
45–54	76.5	68.9
35–44	89.2	83.0
25–34	84.5	85.1
18–24	89.8	88.0
12–17	87.9	80.3
6–11	75.6	71.0
4–5	36.1	26.0

Source: Derived from Table 25, all races, from the National Health Survey [1].

throughout the aging process: (1) the best optical correction and (2) periodic increases in illuminance.

Werner [9] reviewed records of patients aged 25–35 years to quantify the number of symptomatic and asymptomatic changes within two years and within five years of a previous examination. In the total group tested

A Textbook Case

Dr. Leonard Carmichael, former president of Tufts University, liked to apply information from his professional field, psychology. He came late to lunch one day and surprised his companions by announcing grumpily, "Gentlemen, it is not just a textbook maxim that visual discrimination depends upon the level of illumination." He then explained that he'd just had a frustrating bout with a telephone book in an unlighted booth. Even with the aid of a book of paper matches he had been unable to read the number he needed in the telephone book, which was firmly chained inside the booth.

within two years, 15 percent had clinical changes but had no symptoms, and 58 percent had clinical changes with or without symptoms. In the group tested between two and five years of their previous examination, 14 percent had clinical changes but no symptoms, and 54 percent had clinical changes. Werner emphasizes that the large number of asymptomatic patients indicates that regular eye examinations are needed for patients in this age group.

Sperduto [10] presents results of the 1971 to 1972 National Health and Nutrition Examination Survey on the prevalence of myopia in the United States among persons 12 to 54. When persons were classified by the refractive status of the right eye, 25 percent were myopic. Substantially lower rates were found in males than in females, and in Blacks than in Whites. Myopia prevalence rose with family income and educational level. The size of the association of these factors with myopia may result from the link between high income and educational levels with near work, a factor that has been indicted but not convicted of causing myopia.

Contact Lenses

The principle behind contact lenses, like many inventions realized and unrealized, can be traced to Leonardo da Vinci. Like eyeglasses, contact lenses are the result of the efforts of many contributors over the centuries. However, substantial advancements in both the understanding of the principle and the making of contact lenses came in the late nineteenth century. The invention of local anesthetics for the eye in 1884 enabled physicians to fit patients with small, hard, curved lenses resting on the surface of the cornea. Today contact lenses come in hard and soft varieties.

Consumers prefer soft contact lenses because they are easier to fit, more comfortable, and disposable. What is more, they cause less blur when taken out and then switched for spectacles and are adaptable to different lifestyles.

Soft lenses have some disadvantages. They are large and adherent and are removed by direct manipulation with the fingers. They require a strict cleaning regimen and daily sterilization. Soft lenses require more frequent replacement than hard lenses and are more expensive. Many wearers do not comply with the care regimen for contact lenses, and people with dry eyes may not find them suitable.

The majority of refractive errors, such as myopia, hyperopia, and astigmatism, are successfully corrected with contact lenses. Soft lenses now account for 85 percent of all contact lens sales in the United States and 74 percent of all sales worldwide [*11*]. Approximately 24 million people in the United States wear contact lenses. The greatest advantage of contact lenses over spectacles to the myopic individual is the cosmetic and physical relief from thick glasses. For example, the FAA (Federal Aviation Administration) has ruled that "in the performance of aviation duties the use of contact lenses to correct distant visual acuity will not adversely affect safety" and is therefore permissible (as are regular eyeglasses).

The most important feature of contact lenses is that they rest on the surface of the eye. Because of this unique feature, they have numerous potential therapeutic uses that glasses cannot offer. For example, they can be saturated with medication that is then released into the eye, thereby eliminating the need for eyedrops [*4*].

Industrial and Professional Safety

Healthy People 2000 [*12*], a report about the National Health Promotion and Disease Prevention Objectives, estimates that each year 1.3 million people sustain eye injuries. Of these injuries, 1,000 per day or 350,000 per year occur on the job. Over 100,000 of the injuries are permanently disabling. Yet, it is believed that 9 out of 10 injuries could have been prevented had proper eye-safety practices been observed. The report further states that 160,000 school-aged children suffer eye injuries and that 100,000 product-related eye injuries happen in the home every year.

The eye-safety programs that have been established in the workplace have met with various degrees of success. In a study of the high cost paid by industry for preventable eye injuries, John Thackray [*13*] reports that in industrial environments like factories, mines, warehouses, shops and mills, and construction and logging sites, the worker is especially vulnerable to eye injuries. He also explores the obstacles to implementing safety programs, as well as some of the reasons for noncompliance by workers. Thackray points out that in 1980 the National Safety Council reported that 5 percent of all on-the-job injuries were to the eyes. The cost of treating these injuries accounted for $300 million of medical costs in 1983 (well over $500 million in 1991 dollars). The indirect costs, such as time away from work, legal fees, and costs of training new workers, considerably enlarge this figure.

Safety glasses equipped with side shields offer the most protection. Thackray believes that, if employers had a greater awareness of the cost of eye injuries, safety programs would become more common. He also reports that individual workers, unions, and corporations are their own worst enemies in implementing safety programs. Many corporations have initiated eye-safety programs that are ineffective and not enforced. The failure of management to communicate the benefits of eye safety to the workforce is the most cited reason for worker noncompliance. Thackeray would make compliance to eye-safety programs a condition of employment.

Eye-safety measures have had good effect in preventing injuries to athletes. It is estimated that for the year 1980, for example, face protectors for amateur hockey players averted 70,000 eye injuries and saved in excess of $10 million in medical expenses [4].

Eye guards are not the only "protective devices" used in professional life. Visual screening has been used by industry as a tool to direct people away from certain occupations for which they are not visually equipped. An example of an occupation requiring a high level of visual acuity is police work. Police officers must have and maintain high levels of visual skills in order to assess suspects and potentially dangerous situations from both near and far distances. Investigators have deplored [14] the lack of uniform vision standards for police officers and recommended a standard of 20/40 binocular vision as necessary for meeting the requirements of the job. Police shooting statistics [15] indicate that most firearm use occurs within twenty feet of the target and that as a rule sight alignment is not used. Identification of the target is especially critical in deciding whether to shoot.

Good and Augsburger [16] conducted an experiment to find out the proper, uncorrected visual acuity that police applicants should have. They found that the emergency nature of police work requires that police officers must be able to function even if their glasses are knocked off or broken during performance of their duties. The results of their experiment supports the findings of Sheedy and coworkers [15] that 20/40 vision is the necessary standard for police work.

Quality of Life

Poor vision may interfere with daily activities and even cause accidents. Cross-sectional data from the California Department of Motor Vehicles [17] shows a steady rise with age in the proportion of persons having a vision restriction noted on their driving licenses. Among California drivers

Table 11-4. The rank of visual impairment among the leading limiting chronic conditions and rate of occurrence, by sex and age. Respondents report that the visual impairment limits activities and causes disabilities.

	Men		Women	
Age	Rank	Rate/1,000	Rank	Rate/1,000
18–44	4	6	7	3
45–69	10	13	9	12
70–84	5	34	6	35
85+	1	103	2	108

Source: Adapted with permission from Verbrugge [*18*].

26.5 percent have a vision restriction; the percentages range from 13.3 for drivers 16–19 years of age to 88.8 percent for those 90–94 years of age. Without glasses these people would not be allowed to drive.

Corrective lenses permit about one-fourth of the population to drive and are required for them to obtain a driver's license; more serious visual impairment has a considerable impact on a person's whole life. According to Verbrugge [*18*, p. 31], "Disability, not death is the principal consequence of chronic conditions . . . [these conditions] often bother and disable a person for the rest of his or her life." Self-reports obtained from the Health Interview Survey, conducted by the National Center for Health Statistics, indicate that poor vision among adults (persons 18 years of age and older) is a leading chronic condition and a major cause of disability.

With increasing age, visual impairment becomes the leading limiting chronic condition in people's lives (see Table 11-4). Visual impairment affects 11 percent of the population over 55 and is estimated to rank sixth in prevalence and third in impact among disabilities. Although nonfatal, the leading conditions have a large impact on a person's overall well-being and participation in society. Verbrugge [*18*] suggests that because these conditions bother but do not kill, fewer research dollars are spent on eradicating them.

Policy Issues

In reviewing health insurance coverage for visual conditions, we found that eye examinations and applicable treatment for refractive errors come under the classification of "routine" care and thus are not covered by most plans. Gordon and Crooks [19], who surveyed optometric services and private health insurance reimbursement patterns, found that the coverage of eye examinations depends on the diagnosis. The authors emphasize that most health insurance plans do not cover routine or preventive care but reimburse expenses due to disease and eye injury. They further stress the distinction between medical plans and vision plans or riders. When available, vision, eyeglass, or optical plans cover routine eye examinations and ophthalmic materials within specified limits.

As of April 1, 1987, Medicare considers optometrists as physicians, as far as the provision of services they are authorized to perform in accordance with state law or regulation. Medicare covers eye health examinations only when the visit is specifically prompted by a complaint or symptom of eye disease or injury. Routine eye examinations and refractions remain uncovered under Medicare.

Using data from the 1980 National Medical Care Utilization and Expenditure Survey, one group of investigators has reported [20] that minority-group and near-poor children were at highest risk for limited utilization of services and inadequate insurance coverage. Eye examinations and new prescriptions for glasses are examples of services less utilized. Another group reported [21] on results of the Rand Health Insurance Experiment: lower-income enrollees were more adversely affected than higher-income enrollees by enrollment in cost-sharing plans. Free care resulted in improved vision because it increased the frequency of eye examinations and lens purchases.

The U.S. Preventive Services Task Force, whose mission was to evaluate the benefits of early detection and treatment of vision disorders, concluded that there is convincing evidence that early detection and treatment of vision disorders in infants and young children improves the prognosis for normal eye development. In addition, it is widely believed that clinical screening tests can detect vision disorders earlier than parents or teachers can. Other professional organizations, such as the American Academy of Ophthalmology, the American Academy of Pediatrics, the Canadian Task Force, and the American Optometric Association, recommend annual screening of schoolchildren up to 6 years of age for visual acuity and ocular alignment; they also recommend screening, with lower frequency, for persons up to 40 years old. Thereafter, annual examinations are recommended.

Milne [22] examined 213 men and 272 women aged 63–90 years in Edinburgh. Worsening of visual acuity occurred over five years in 12 percent of men and 14 percent of women; improvement was noted in 15 percent of men and 10 percent of women. The change is insidious; people do not realize that they are gradually losing acuity and so do not get new corrective lenses. Simply asking a person being tested "Has your eyesight changed since you were last here?" was not satisfactory in identifying change in visual acuity. Similarly, Stone and Shannon [23], in a survey of middle-aged persons from a general practice, found that replies to the question "Do you have difficulty in seeing distant objects?" were poor identifiers of visual impairment. Thus, older adults usually do not detect changes in their vision themselves, and up to 25 percent of the elderly may be using an incorrect lens prescription [24].

Conclusion

Nearly everyone at some stage of life will need correction of a refractive error. Not much can be done to prevent the loss of visual acuity that occurs with normal aging, but there is great comfort in knowing that treatment for the problem, glasses or contact lenses, is readily available, effective, and relatively inexpensive. Although refractive errors such as myopia or hyperopia are not life-threatening conditions, they can, when left unattended, reduce one's participation in recreational and social activities and narrow one's occupational possibilities.

Because loss in visual acuity is not readily detected by the loser, regular visual checkups are needed as part of routine health care, with changes in prescriptions as needed. And because not everyone experiences the same gradual visual loss at the same time, frequency of testing for visual acuity should be dependent on age and rate of visual loss.

Preventing occupational eye injuries seems to require better appreciation of the value of eye-safety programs by workers, unions, and employers. Better dissemination of the benefits of routine prevention and more training to instill protective habits can maintain advances already achieved by eye-safety programs and improve their total effectiveness. The huge benefits of protective eyewear in sports have already been documented.

Society is fortunate that visual handicaps can so often and so readily be ameliorated.

Editors' Note

Although it is easy for a person to perceive the difference that lenses make when prescriptions are being changed, studies show that people do not notice their gradual loss of vision. Nor do parents and teachers recognize changes in the vision of children in their care very well. Consequently, periodic eye examinations are needed for almost everyone.

Lenses are needed by nearly everyone at some time. They improve quality of life by extending a person's ability to perform in some occupations, to drive, to read, and to participate in social and recreational events. Yet despite the great difference lenses can make at a relatively low cost, low-income groups are frequently denied access to appropriate vision care. This is so because Medicare and ordinary health insurance policies do not cover routine eye examinations, and because cost-sharing reduces purchases of lenses by the poor.

Use of safety lenses is less than optimal also, but for different reasons. Safety glasses preserve quality of life by preventing the eye injuries that can occur in dangerous occupations and in sports. Yet often they are not used merely because of negligence. Especially in workplaces, education and enforcement of use of safety glasses is needed.

12

Dentistry

ALEXIA ANTCZAK-BOUCKOMS
AND J. F. C. TULLOCH

Background

Dentistry has contributed to improved oral health and quality of life by developing treatments that prevent tooth decay and restore diseased teeth in form, function, and appearance. In this century, fluoride more than any other factor has led to these improvements. Fluoride has eliminated the nightmare of toothaches and dental infections for millions of children and has changed the expectation among adults that tooth loss is inevitable. In addition, there have been technical developments in materials, equipment, and services in the profession. These two trends—prevention and restoration—have worked together to dramatically improve oral health.

In this chapter, we summarize data on the need for and use of dental services. To illustrate the impact of prevention and new restorative treatments on patients' lives since the early 1900s, we describe the experiences of four generations of a family. The people are fictitious and are to be taken as illustrative of their particular generations.

Four Generations

Elizabeth, born in 1985, benefits most from the decline in dental decay and the improvement in technologies. Like the majority of her peers (94 percent of 6-year-olds), she has not developed any cavities that need filling and she may never do so [1]. Exposure to fluoride—systemically, while the teeth are developing, or topically, after they have erupted—has substantially reduced her risk for cavities [2]. As Elizabeth's teeth are forming, ingested fluoride, from fluoridated water or supplemental tablets, is incorporated into the tooth enamel. This provides a protective effect against tooth decay throughout life. Once her teeth erupt, topical exposure to fluoride in the drinking water, in fluoride rinses, and in toothpastes provide added resistance to decay [3].

Elizabeth also benefits by having had her back teeth sealed. Teeth are sealed by filling the grooves of the biting surfaces with a plastic material that prevents bacteria from causing decay. If she does develop a cavity, it is likely to be small and detected early. In addition, the materials now available to restore cavities generally do not require as much drilling as was necessary in the past. Hence these fillings should be both less painful to place and less likely to weaken the remaining tooth. Should Elizabeth develop cavities in her front teeth or fracture a front tooth in an accident, tooth-colored materials can be used to restore those teeth more conservatively than in the past with minimal or no drilling.

Disease trends and innovations have been so rapid in the past twenty years that it is instructive to consider Elizabeth's Uncle Bill, born 22 years earlier in 1963. Uncle Bill benefited from the widespread introduction of fluoride to public water supplies in the 1960s and 1970s. Public water fluoridation was introduced in 1945, and by 1989 fluoridated water was available to 130 million people in the United States [4], or approximately 50 percent of the U.S. population. It is unlikely that further efforts to expand water fluoridation will substantially increase the proportion of the population drinking fluoridated water, as 42 of the 50 largest cities are already fluoridated. Additional efforts would have to be aimed at comparatively small cities or municipalities and would result in relatively modest increases in the population served. Although Uncle Bill grew up drinking water that was fluoridated and had frequent fluoride treatments from his dentist, he did not use daily fluoride mouthrinses, nor were dental sealants available. He has developed a handful of small cavities that have been filled with silver amalgam. These fillings are likely to need replacement during his lifetime due to material breakdown, but, because they are small, they should not compromise the function or life expectancy of his teeth. Barring trauma due to accidents, he is unlikely to need extensive restorative dental treatments such as root canals, crowns, bridges, dentures, or implants.

Elizabeth's mother and Elizabeth's aunts and other uncles, born between 1947 and 1954, although siblings of Uncle Bill, have very different dental histories. They were not exposed to fluoride as children and have experienced considerable dental decay. All have large silver amalgam fillings in virtually all of their back teeth, some gold or porcelain crowns, and at least some teeth requiring removal of the nerve through root canal treatment. Although Elizabeth's aunts and uncles are all fortunate enough not to have lost any teeth because of caries yet, many of their peers have, and they are still at risk for such loss. Two percent of this age group are missing all of their teeth (are edentulous), while the remaining 98 percent are missing a mean of 4 teeth out of 28 [5]. Their large fillings require periodic replacement, often with a larger or more complex restoration. Sometimes replacement causes nerve damage, necessitating root canal treatment and crowns. They will likely need restorative services for the rest of their lives and will benefit from the technological advances of the past twenty years. Although they are at risk of losing some teeth, their risk of losing all their teeth is small.

Elizabeth's grandparents, born between 1918 and 1929, did not benefit from fluoride in any form. They have experienced considerable dental disease and pose the most complicated restorative problems. To illustrate the impact of dental caries on this and older generations, the most common reason for rejecting recruits from the military in both World Wars I and II was dental decay. Although many of the grandparents' generation (42 percent) have no natural teeth remaining, the mean number of missing teeth for this cohort is 10 of 28 [5].

Traditionally, the treatments available to this group are fixed bridges, when a few teeth are missing, or removable partial dentures, when a greater number are missing. Only recently have dental implants been available to provide an alternative to these two replacements. Implants are metal posts inserted into the jawbone that can be used to replace single missing teeth or serve as anchors for fixed bridges that replace several teeth. Although implants require a surgical procedure for insertion, are associated with a risk of failure, and are expensive, they appear to offer esthetic, functional, and psychological advantages not previously available. Because they are anchored in the jawbone like natural teeth, they feel, look, and function better than dentures.

Elizabeth's grandparents' generation has benefited late in life from greater access to dental services, improved restorative materials and technical procedures, and changes in philosophy of treatment. The availability of antibiotics, analgesics, and aseptic technique fostered a shift toward more conservative treatment. The introduction of radiographs allowed earlier detection of disease, and with root canal therapy, teeth with advanced dental decay extending into the nerve could be saved.

Elizabeth's great-grandparents, born before the turn of the century, probably lost all their teeth early in their lives and could expect only poor

Mean decayed, missing, or
filled surfaces per person

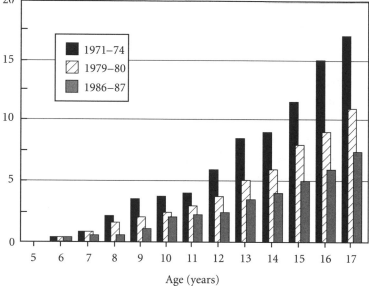

Figure 12-1. Changes in mean decayed, missing, or filled surfaces in permanent teeth, by age. (Data from National Center for Health Statistics, National Health and Nutrition Examination Survey 1971–1973; National Institute of Dental Research, National Survey of the Oral Health of U.S. Children Aged 5–17, 1979–1980; and National Survey of the Oral Health of U.S. Children Aged 5–17, 1986–1987.)

prosthetic replacements of their missing teeth. In the early 1900s materials used to fabricate full dentures were not very successful, and dentures were uncomfortable and ugly. In some cases these dentures caused severe tissue irritation and even precancerous changes. This generation had very limited access to preventive dental services and thus experienced significant dental disease. Furthermore, dentists in those days generally recommended the early extraction of even mildly diseased teeth to prevent potentially life-threatening infectious complications of dental disease [6].

Figures 12-1 and 12-2 help illustrate these changes across generations. The difference in risk of disease between Uncle Bill and his siblings, separated only by ten years of age, is due to the introduction of water fluoridation. Figure 12-1, reporting results of three national surveys spanning sixteen years, supports the conclusion that this is not an age effect but a cohort effect. If it were an age effect, Uncle Bill would have fewer

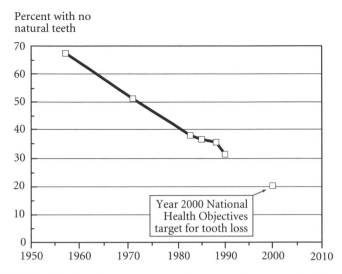

Figure 12-2. Decline in the percentage of persons 65 years and older with no natural teeth, selected years. (Data from the National Center for Health Statistics, cited in Burt and Ekland [2, pp. 84, 244].)

lesions simply because he is so much younger than his siblings and would catch up with them as he grew older. However, this figure demonstrates that although rates of cavity formation increase with age, for each survey there has been a decrease in the rate across all age groups. For example, consider the right-most group of bars, for children age 17. In 1972, the mean number of damaged surfaces was 17, in 1979, about 11, and in 1986, about 7.5—a reduction of 35 percent in the first 7 years, and of 32 percent in the next 7 years. In addition, over the 3 survey periods the rate of increase in cavities with age is less, and this trend is expected to continue.

Figure 12-2 summarizes the change in percentage of people 65 years of age and older with no natural teeth from 1957 to 1990. There has been a steady and dramatic decline in those who are toothless, and the trend is expected to continue. The Year 2000 National Health Objectives for tooth loss has set an edentulous rate of 20 percent as the target.

The Continuing Demand for Restorative Services

In spite of the dramatic decline in disease in the past thirty years, a substantial demand for restorative dental services remains. In the United States, 96 percent of adults between the ages of 18 and 65 have one or more carious or filled teeth [5]. More than 200 million fillings are placed each year, and general-practice dentists spend at least 50 percent of their time on restorative care. Without these services, carious lesions and tooth loss can result in pain and disability that affect work productivity [7], leisure activities, social functioning (including speech), and appearance.

The National Institute of Dental Research recently reported that 50 percent of American schoolchildren aged 5 to 17 are now caries-free in their permanent teeth [1]. This still leaves approximately 18 million children with caries requiring treatment, however. In addition, of the 17-year-old population group, 84 percent have at least one filling already, suggesting a continued future risk in this cohort. The segment of the population aged 18–64 years in the National Survey of Adults of 1985–1986 had an average of 10 decayed, missing, or filled teeth [5].

Dentists anticipate a large increase in need for restorative dental services among the population 65 years and older during the next few decades. Given current population projections, the number of teeth at risk for dental disease in this age group in 1980 was 2.8 billion and is expected to increase to 5 billion teeth at risk by 2020. This group was born before the current decline in caries. Thus many of their remaining teeth have already been restored, and these fillings will need replacement. In addition, 63 percent of the elderly and 21 percent of the population aged 18–64 have root caries, decay on the root surface of the teeth. Root caries has only recently been recognized as a significant clinical problem, now that many elderly are retaining their teeth longer. In previous cohorts teeth were lost at such a young age that there was not enough time for them to develop gum recession and thus be at risk for root caries. The decline in restorative treatment needs in the under-20 age group has been offset to some extent by the increased need in the adult and elderly population.

Interventions

In 1990, $34 billion was spent on dental services in the United States, or approximately 5 percent of all national health expenditures [8]. Access to dental services has continually increased, for a number of reasons [2]. First, there has been an increase in the number of dentists and auxiliaries providing services. Dental schools in the 1970s expanded enrollment in response to government concerns about an undersupply. Second, there has been an increase in productivity in dental practices, as a result of technological developments such as the high-speed dental drill and composite restorative materials. Finally, more people have sought dental care over the past three decades because of socioeconomic factors. These include increased discretionary income and the increased availability of third-party payment for dental services. For example, in 1957–58 only 37 percent of the population reported visiting a dentist during the preceding twelve months, but in 1986 57 percent did so [2]. As recently as 1970, over 90 percent of dental expenditures were paid out of pocket; with the rise in private dental insurance as a benefit of employment, however, currently only about 55 percent of expenditures are paid by the patient.

Although access to dental services has increased in general in the United States, for important segments of the population it has not. The poor and members of certain racial and ethnic minorities use dental services much less frequently, and they are more likely to use emergency services and less likely to use preventive services than the rest of the population [9]. Some 60 percent of dental decay occurs in 20 percent of the population, mostly in these underserved groups. Especially at risk are children who are from families with lower incomes or unemployed parents, who are non-White, who are infected with the cariogenic bacterium *Streptococcus mutans,* and who have poor toothbrushing habits. Native American children are at particular risk for the development of Baby Bottle Tooth Decay, which results when infants fall asleep while still sucking on bottles filled with sugary drinks. Among the homeless, 97 percent need dental care but are not eligible for coverage under Medicaid. In states that include dental services as a benefit under Medicaid, reimbursement is generally at a level so far below community averages that many eligible patients are unable to find providers willing to treat them. Even though there is perceived excess capacity in the dental care system and wide availability of dental insurance, not all in need of dental treatment seek care. Treatment decisions are influenced by factors such as the extent of the decay, the number of teeth needing repair or replacement, whether the restoration will be visible, treatment philosophies, patient preferences, and cost factors, including who will pay.

When a tooth is damaged or deformed, it can generally be restored in one visit with some type of plastic material, which hardens after being placed in the tooth. These include silver amalgam, tooth-colored composite materials, and various cements. When a tooth is more severely affected, such that plastic materials are no longer suitable, it is frequently necessary to cover the tooth with a cast-gold or porcelain-fused-to-metal restoration. These procedures require more than one office visit and the assistance of a laboratory, which considerably increases the cost. (See Table 12-1.)

Table 12-1. Classification scheme for restorative needs.

1. Tooth restoration
   a. Minor—silver amalgams, tooth-colored composite materials
   b. Major—silver amalgams, porcelain-fused-to-metal crowns, full gold crowns

2. Tooth replacement
   a. Single—fixed bridge, implants
   b. Multiple—fixed bridge, removable partial denture, complete denture, implants

Missing teeth can be replaced with bridges or removable partial dentures. These alternatives involve laboratory procedures and relatively high costs. Traditionally, when bridges are made, the teeth on either side of the missing tooth (teeth) are crowned to serve as anchors for the bridge. Preparation for the crown requires that a considerable amount of tooth substance be removed, with some resultant trauma to these teeth. Newer materials have allowed more conservative preparations to be used.

When considering the benefits of restorative dentistry, we must also consider the ill effects that may result from these services. These include potential toxic effects of the materials, mechanical injury from the restoration, weakening of the tooth from drilling, and the risk of caries recurrence due to imperfect materials and techniques. Once placed, dental materials are in prolonged contact with living tissues. Although they are made as strong and inert as possible, materials do deteriorate, and minute amounts of component substances may be released into the mouth and pose some theoretical health risk.

Amalgams

Silver amalgam has been used to restore teeth for 150 years. The safety and efficacy of various formulations have been tested in clinical trials, and the benefits of this material for restoring tooth structure and function are universally acknowledged. It is relatively inert, strong, and durable. It is comparatively inexpensive and easily manipulated, which is an advantage both for immediate placement by the dentist and for the speed with which the tooth becomes functional again.

Recent public concern regarding the safety of amalgam fillings followed reports that minute amounts of mercury vapor are released during chewing. Also, cases of patients with systemic complaints reporting immediate relief from symptoms after removal of amalgam fillings has heightened interest in this topic. However, a National Institutes of Health Technology

Assessment Conference, The Effects and Side Effects of Dental Restorative Materials, concluded that current evidence does not indicate that silver amalgam fillings pose a risk to human health.

The case reports of symptom relief following amalgam removal were not substantiated with medical documentation. In addition, it has been demonstrated that removal of amalgam fillings causes mercury vapor release and that the total body burden of mercury is relatively high after filling removal. If these patients experienced relief of symptoms immediately following filling removal, it was in the presence of mercury levels much higher than the levels that would result from leaching from silver amalgams in normal function. Therefore, chronic mercury exposure from dental amalgams is not likely to have been the cause of their systemic symptoms. Without this material, it is quite probable that most persons aged 40 and over would be completely, or nearly completely, toothless.

Silver amalgam has been used to restore the vast majority of all dental decay for several generations, but it is likely that amalgam will be replaced in the near future, following the introduction of improved composite resins. These resins will offer better appearances than amalgam and will eliminate any concerns about the theoretical health risks posed by the presence of mercury in silver amalgams.

Esthetic Restorations

In response to esthetic concerns, dentists developed materials in the 1960s that have revolutionized restoration of anterior teeth. Because only a minimum of drilling is required by the new methods, these innovations reduce trauma to the tooth nerve. The tooth enamel is made porous with a mild acid, to strengthen the bond of the composite material to the tooth. Teeth can be restored, often without local anesthesia, in a single office visit. These restorations are very attractive and comparatively inexpensive.

Prior to the development of these composite restorations, the alternative was to crown the tooth. In such cases, a significant amount of the tooth had to be removed to allow the crown to be placed. This process entails several visits to the dentist and considerable cost. The cost for a single crown ranges from $400 to $1,000, and crowns usually require replacement at some time between 10 and 20 years later.

Endodontic Therapy

In the 1960s methods were developed to remove damaged nerve tissue from teeth with deep cavities or large fractures. This has provided the tremendous benefit of maintaining teeth that otherwise would have been lost. Improved antiseptic and radiographic techniques, as well as a better understanding of wound healing, helped make maintenance of teeth without vital nerves successful and routine. The ability to "save" teeth with root canal treatment even when the vitality of the nerve has been lost has contributed to the shift in treatment philosophy leading to fewer extractions and more conservative restoration. Although many people think of root canal treatment as painful, this impression is unjustified, given current techniques and anesthetic methods.

Dental Implants

Interest in dental implants, artificial replacements of missing teeth that are permanently anchored in the jawbone, is long-standing. Evidence exists that Egyptians placed precious stones and metals and that Mayans inserted teeth carved from seashells into jawbones where teeth were lost. Although more recent attempts to develop dental implants began in the 1940s, little success was achieved until the 1980s, when biocompatible materials and techniques for integrating the implant into the bone were developed.

Dental implants present a special opportunity to consider quality-of-life issues in restorative dentistry. In 1992, an estimated 300,000 implants were placed in the United States. This procedure marks a dramatic improvement in dentistry's effectiveness: implants offer a very appealing alternative to the traditional methods for replacement of teeth. For many patients, prior to implants, the sequel to tooth loss was the embarrassment of loose-fitting dentures.

Implants may be used to replace teeth missing for a variety of reasons. Although tooth loss due to dental disease is rapidly declining, rates of loss due to trauma (car accidents, for example, or hockey pucks) are not likely to decline. Future rates of trauma to teeth will depend on the distribution and use of protective equipment such as face masks, seat belts, and, perhaps, airbags.

The potential demand for this restorative technology over the next 10–20 years is substantial, given the large proportion of older persons missing some or all of their teeth, but several factors may militate against this potential demand. First, rates of tooth loss are more cohort-dependent than age-dependent. The next generation of persons to reach the over-55 age group will have lost far fewer teeth than the elders of today. Second, not all sites where teeth are missing are suitable for implants, and many systemic and local factors may preclude their use. The final factor that limits utilization is the very high cost. A diagnostic workup often involves a CAT (Computed Axial Tomography) scan and/or MRI (Magnetic Resonance Imaging). The base of the implant is usually placed during one surgical procedure. Then, after the bone heals, the implant is uncovered during a second surgery to attach a post that can be used to anchor a restoration above the gum line. In addition, interim restorative procedures (removable partial dentures) may be needed. Thus, a single tooth replacement may range in cost from $1,000 to $3,000, while more extensive replacement of several missing teeth can easily cost $30,000.

Lessons for the Future

Public health, private practice, and personal care have all contributed to a substantial and continuing decline in the rate and severity of dental decay over the past few decades. In concert with this decline, improvements in materials and techniques have contributed to a shift in philosophy toward more conservative approaches to treatment. In many instances treatment can be rendered faster, with less pain, and at lower relative cost than in the past. In addition, technological advances such as dental implants provide new opportunities for treatment and improved quality of life. Although disease rates are declining, demand for services has increased because of economic and social changes that have improved access to dental services for a large proportion of the population. Expectations of what dentistry can do have also risen. Table 12-2 traces the important dates in the history of modern innovations in dentistry. In the early 1900s the rejection of so many recruits for World War I because of dental decay focused attention on the poor oral health of the population. This coincided with a general belief in the theory of focal infection in medicine, which stated that a site of local disease, such as a decayed tooth, could be responsible for a large number of systemic disorders.

Three developments in this century have had the most dramatic and lasting impact on oral health. They are the introduction of local anesthetics and antibiotics, water fluoridation, and improved personal oral hygiene. They have changed both the patient's perception of dental care and the profession's philosophy of treatment. Because of local anesthetics, dental treatment is no longer limited by the pain tolerance of the patient. With attention to antiseptic technique and the use of antibiotics, many teeth

Table 12-2. Important events and technologies in the history of dental health.

1910–1920	World War I (recruits rejected for dental health problems)
1920–1930	Gies Report on Dental Education Dental Act for Licensure of Dentists
1940–1950	World War II (recruits still rejected for dental health problems) Local anesthetics First public water fluoridation
1950–1960	High-speed drills
1960–1970	Health Professions Education Act Sealants Plaque-control programs
1970–1980	Acid-etch technique Rise in dental insurance
1980–1990	NIH Consensus Conference on Dental Sealants NIH Consensus Conference on Dental Implants NIH Technology Assessment Conference on Restorative Dental Materials

with infections of the nerve or surrounding gum and bone can be treated and the teeth retained, rather than extracted to prevent life-threatening infections. The introduction of fluoride in the drinking water has not only decreased the dental decay rate but has also spurred a new orientation toward prevention of dental disease. Although concerns have been raised about the safety of fluoride, all hypothesized adverse effects have been without empirical support. Finally, a greater availability of toothpaste, toothbrushes, and dental floss, along with increased commercial advertising of these products, has resulted in improved personal oral hygiene.

Several technical developments in the second half of this century have made important contributions to dental health. First, the introduction of high-speed drills has made restorative treatment faster and less painful. The new technology made treatment less onerous for the patient and increased the productivity of the dentist. Second, the introduction of plastic tooth-colored materials and acid-etching for bonding improved the effectiveness of sealants and made it possible to repair damaged front teeth with minimal drilling. Finally, the development of biocompatible materials made dental implants possible.

Although dentistry has made great strides in preventing and treating oral diseases, one cannot ignore the residual impact of oral diseases on the population: not only are 21 million work-days lost annually because of dental disease [7], but, in spite of dramatic decreases in rates of dental caries, the majority of the population still experiences some need for services each year. Preventive technologies, with the exception of fluoride, have been grossly underutilized. While there is evidence that oral health promotion and prevention are effective, many of these technologies have not been adequately put into practice [10]. Dental sealants provide a dramatic example of how preventive techniques are not always adequately transferred into practice. Ninety-five percent of all dental caries in U.S. children is on the biting surfaces of back teeth, the type of cavity sealants were developed to prevent. Yet a survey of U.S. schoolchildren in 1986–87 found that only 8 percent of those aged 5–17 had any sealants on their teeth. This technology could virtually eliminate the residual dental decay in the United States, yet it is barely being used.

Simply proving that this preventive technique works has not ensured utilization. It is neither the concept of prevention nor the technical difficulty of using the technology that poses a barrier to use, however. Dentists and consumers appear to believe in the potential for prevention in dentistry. Many people seek regular preventive treatment from dentists when they have their teeth cleaned or have fluoride treatments. Similarly, it is not likely that a technical barrier holds back the use of sealants, as the techniques for sealants are identical to those used for tooth-colored fillings for front teeth. Introduced at the same time, these filling materials are universally used by dentists and demanded by patients. In fact, many dentists no longer use silver amalgam but rely solely on these composites for all restorative needs.

To increase the use of sealants, dentists must make patients aware of the availability and effectiveness of this technology. Very recently, insurance coverage for sealants has become more widespread, and there is evidence that this has increased their use.

The potential exists for problems with dental caries to increase as the population ages and retains more teeth. Further, many medical conditions and medications can reduce saliva production and cause dry mouth. When saliva, which normally acts to protect teeth from decay, is decreased, the risk of decay increases. Thus far, some 250 medications have been shown to cause dry mouth.

As already noted, expectations of what dentistry can do have risen. Early in this century, dental treatment was sought only for relief of pain (via tooth extraction) and for replacement of teeth with dentures. Now, many patients seek regular preventive care and expect esthetic perfection. Discolored or chipped teeth are bonded and crooked teeth are straightened, even in adulthood. Fear of pain no longer deters many people from visiting the dentist, because of the universal and very effective use of analgesics and anesthetics. In fact, the decline in caries rate, the use of adequate analgesia, and the incorporation of behavior management techniques have resulted in a generation of children who look forward to regular dental visits.

Editors' Note

Improvements in dental health are well illustrated by the reduction in the percent of people 65 years and older who have no teeth. In the late 1950s the percent was about 69, but by 1990 it was about 31, and it is anticipated that by the year 2000 less than 20 percent will have no natural teeth. Currently half the children aged 5–17 years are caries-free. Fluoride in water and dental rinses and toothpaste have reduced the rate of caries drastically (though there is room to improve this record by fluoridating water in more places). Sealants have the potential to reduce the rate even further. Though they are rarely heralded, the effects of these treatments on dental disease are as spectacular as the effects of vaccines on infectious diseases can be.

Among the other advances mentioned in this chapter are the reduction in pain experienced by the dental patient, which has helped to reduce the avoidance of dental care; new materials and new methods for restoring lost teeth; and an increase in the coverage of dental services by health insurance. These improvements are reflected in the continuing improvements in dental health documented by various health surveys. Though there is room for improvement—in greater education and more insurance coverage for more people—dentistry offers many examples of technological innovation at high quality and reasonable price.

PART G

Quality of Life and Cost-Effectiveness

Nearly normal joint mobility and relief of pain can now be offered to individuals with incapacitating osteoarthritis of knee and hip. This benefit can be achieved at a surgical risk that many sufferers are willing to assume, even well beyond age 65. Because osteoarthritis is almost never a cause of death, the benefit being sought is an improvement in quality of life, usually in the form of pain relief and improved joint function.

A clinical trial of joint replacement poses special problems in design—blinding the subject and observer to the treatment, for example, or quantifying changes in pain. Nevertheless, credible assessments of joint replacement have been carried out. In addition, they call attention to another aspect of evaluation: how outcomes are valued. For instance, treatment is expensive but enhances function, often with striking success. Economists and other evaluators would like to credit the procedure with recapturing some of society's financial investment, and the "return on the investment" is traditionally measured in the form of the patient's increased capacity to be economically productive, to work. Although the ability to live without nursing or housekeeping care can appropriately be included in the calculation, the age of those receiving treatment and policies regarding age of retirement mean that few patients will re-enter the work force. The societal decision about whether to offer joint replacement to the elderly will have to be made on the basis of improvements in an individual's quality of life rather than economic gains for the society as a whole.

13

Total Joint Replacement for the Treatment of Osteoarthritis

JENNIFER F. TAYLOR AND ELISABETH BURDICK

Background

Many different diseases lead to arthritis (literally, inflammation of the joints), but the most common variety—osteoarthritis—is associated with a metabolic remodeling of the joints and wear and tear on the joints from use. Osteoarthritis becomes more frequent with advancing age and with excessive use of the affected joints. It is characterized by loss of cartilage from the joint surfaces and overgrowth of bone at the joints. When the cartilage no longer cushions the movement of bone over bone in the joint, pain, deformity, and loss of mobility follow. The joints most commonly affected are the knee and hip, because these are the main weight-bearing joints of the body. In the interests of simplicity in this chapter, we will use the more general term *arthritis* to refer to the specific condition of osteoarthritis.

Those afflicted with arthritis may be unable to work or perform household tasks without pain. For patients with unremitting pain and severe limitations of mobility, orthopedic surgery offers many options, including the replacement of segments of bone, sections of the knee, or total joint replacement (arthroplasty). In this chapter we focus on one treatment, total knee and hip replacement for the treatment of arthritis in older persons (over age 60), and provide an overview of the burden arthritis imposes on both the individual and society, the benefits and risks of joint replacement, and associated health policy issues. A composite but fictitious case illustrates the typical experience of a patient with arthritis of the knee.

Patients at Risk and Their Symptoms

Approximately 15.8 million Americans age 25–74 have signs of arthritis. Of these, an estimated 80 percent experience some degree of pain, instability, or limited range of motion of the affected joints. The remaining 20 percent are severely restricted and are unable to perform major activities of daily living. Arthritis leads to 46 million physician visits and 68 million lost work-days annually [2].

The incidence of arthritis in men increases steadily with aging. Women have an abrupt increase after the menopause, and then the incidence of joint disease tends to level off. Seventy percent more middle-aged women than men have arthritis of the hip, though among the most elderly men and women, the rates are comparable. The knee is three times more commonly affected than the hip [2]. Rates of arthritis of the knee among men increase until roughly age 80. Rates of knee-joint disease in women are stable from approximately ages 50 through 79, at an incidence of just less than 1,000 per 100,000 person-years [2].

Pain and physical limitations are the leading complaints of patients with arthritis. Patients often report difficulty in rising from a chair, walking, going up or down stairs, as well as difficulty, due to chronic joint pain and fatigue, in performing work or engaging in social and sexual activities. These symptoms are associated with negative self-image, depression, and anxiety [3].

Arthritis has no cure. Physicians may prescribe pain medication or non-weight-bearing exercises to maintain mobility and strengthen muscles surrounding the affected joints. With increasing severity, however, a small minority of patients become unable to work, to provide self-care, or to live independently. They may require the assistance of canes or walkers, or even wheelchairs, and live with unrelenting pain. Replacement of the affected joints may provide the most satisfactory relief for these patients.

Total Joint Replacement Surgery

From the time of the first published report of hip replacement in 1860, the field of orthopedic surgery has witnessed changes in surgical technique, prosthetic design, and prosthetic materials. Artificial joints have been manufactured from a variety of substances: wood, ivory, rubber, glass, and state-of-the-art metals, plastics, and ceramics.

In hip arthroplasty, the surgeon removes the rounded top of the femur, or thigh bone, which fits into the joint socket in the pelvic bone, and replaces it with a metal, plastic, or ceramic prosthesis implanted into the femur for stability. In knee arthroplasty, the surgeon replaces the entire knee joint connected above to the femur and below to the tibia. According to the Arthritis Foundation [4], replacement surgery for knees and hips results in the reduction or elimination of pain and restoration of mobility in an estimated 95 percent of cases.

A 1991 study [5] estimated the annual number of joint replacement operations at 60.8 per 100,000 people in 1983–1986; this figure represents an increase over the reported rate of 20.5 per 100,000 in 1971–1974. The increasing number of total joint replacements probably does not reflect an increase in the overall incidence of joint disease, but rather the increased availability of the surgery itself [5]. And as availability has increased, the proportion of older persons electing to undergo joint replacement increased, as has the number of older people.

Case Vignette: Joint Replacement

William is a retired carpet layer who had arthritis in both knees. Before his knee arthroplasty, eight years ago at age 64, he was in constant pain. He was unable to go grocery shopping, work in his garden, or play with his grandchildren. Because he could no longer climb stairs or do routine home maintenance, he had to move to a seniors' community. After several discussions with his orthopedist, William decided to undergo bilateral total knee replacement.

William's case followed an average postoperative course. Within three days after his surgery, William began walking with assistance and started some limited physical therapy. He was discharged from the hospital thirteen days after his surgery and continued to see a physical therapist for approximately five months after his knees were replaced. Now, at age 72, his gait is normal and he experiences slight pain only during strenuous exercise.

William has resumed an active social life and is able to spend time with his children and grandchildren free from crippling pain and physical limitations. Currently his x-rays show no signs of prosthetic loosening or excessive wear. He has not experienced severe pain or infection of bone or soft tissue, as sometimes occurs after replacement surgery.

Recovery and Rehabilitation

A study of 102 patients who underwent knee replacement showed that the average hospital stay following surgery was 10.2 days [6]. In a separate study of 119 unilateral or bilateral total hip replacements performed on a single day or in two stages, the average hospital stay was 9 days for patients who underwent unilateral hip replacement, 15 days for patients who underwent bilateral hip replacement on the same day, and 19 days for patients who underwent bilateral two-stage hip replacement [7].

Recently, the customary postoperative course has changed from immobilization to a program of immediate mobilization using a continuous passive motion machine [5]. This machine exercises the replaced joints without active assistance by the patient. Immediate mobilization facilitates wound healing, decreases swelling, and may reduce hospital stays through more rapid rehabilitation. Some researchers found that the cost of using continuous passive motion during rehabilitation, compared with the cost of standard rehabilitation alone, is lower [6].

Complications

Although total joint replacement is associated with low mortality and improved quality of life, arthroplasty poses some risks. The primary complications are infection and deep-vein thrombosis (the formation of blood clots in the large veins of the legs and pelvis). With appropriate patient care, these risks can be reduced and treated effectively.

Infection in the area surrounding the implant is the most severe complication of joint replacement. The incidence of infection ranges from 1.1 to 12.4 percent [8]. The rate of infection among 3,000 primary, total knee replacements at the Mayo Clinic was 1.2 percent. Investigators report the highest rates of serious infection (11.8 percent) among patients with previous surgery around the hip joint [9]. Other patients at greater risk for infection include those with skin ulcers or compromised immune function.

To reduce the risk of infection, antibiotics are administered both before and after surgery. Some implant types are also impregnated with antibiotics as an added prophylaxis against infection. And, indeed, infection rates have decreased over the past several decades because of the increased use of prophylactic antibiotics, improved surgical techniques, and improved prosthetic design. For example, implants have decreased in size but increased in strength and flexibility. Implanting smaller prostheses generally requires a smaller surgical incision. The wound heals faster and its smaller surface area permits fewer bacteria to enter, further reducing the likelihood of serious infection.

The second complication of joint replacement is thrombosis, or excessive blood clotting within blood vessels, particularly veins. Thrombosis is a significant risk for patients undergoing total joint replacement. When one of these clots forms in a vein, fragments may break off and travel to the lungs as a pulmonary embolus. The risk of thromboembolic disease is compounded by patient age and lowered mobility, as well as the site, extent, nature, and duration of the operative procedure [10].

Pulmonary embolism occurs at rates of 2–16 percent, with mortality rates of 0.3–3.4 percent [10], making this complication the most common cause of death for postsurgical total hip replacement patients. To reduce this risk, physicians administer preventive treatment with anticoagulants. In a sample of 638 patients who underwent total knee replacement, deep-vein thrombosis developed in 84 percent of untreated patients. In comparison, the rate of thrombosis among patients who received prophylactic treatment was 57 percent [11].

Success and Complications in the Very Elderly

The age range of patients receiving arthroplasty increasingly includes the very elderly, despite their higher risk of associated surgical complications. A study of 107 arthroplasty patients over age 80 between 1978 and 1985 found that patients over 80 had more complications than younger patients, including higher operative mortality [12]. However, 75 percent of the patients achieved satisfactory outcomes, which included substantial pain relief as measured by the Harris hip score. The Harris hip score provides a single measure of various medical aspects of the hip, such as pain, function, range of motion, and deformity.

The postoperative course for older patients is also more complicated than that for younger patients. The patients over age 80 in this study had longer hospital stays (37 days, on average), more surgical complications, including thromboembolic episodes and heart attack, and higher rates of femoral fracture and hip dislocation. Because of the satisfactory results obtained in a majority of patients, however, the number of arthroplasties offered to the very elderly is likely to continue to increase despite more frequent and protracted complications.

After Arthroplasty

Even after the successful completion of postoperative rehabilitation, arthroplasty patients must be followed because the prosthetic devices can and do wear out and the patients may require a second operation to replace the device. The Mayo Clinic has compiled data on the outcomes of replacement surgery, the Total Joint Registry, that includes information such as the patient's age, sex, and underlying diagnosis, type of implant, duration of operation, complications, and reoperations. Rand and Ilstrup [13] used it to analyze the survival of 9,200 total knee arthroplasties performed on 5,810 patients at the Mayo Clinic between 1971 and 1987. They found that patient age over 60 was associated with a higher level of prosthetic survival. Higher activity levels in younger patients may explain why their ten-year prosthetic survival rates are 6 percent lower, 82 percent versus 76 percent, than those for older patients.

Economic Benefits

As we have seen in earlier chapters, analysts may use a variety of methods to evaluate the merit of a medical intervention. Surgical joint replacement can be assessed on the basis of pain relief, improved mobility and function, and overall risk. Any thoroughgoing evaluation will also include an assessment of the stream of financial benefits recovered by an intervention. An example would be the earning power from employment that might be restored by improvement in joint function resulting from surgery. Although simple in principle, such economic evaluations are often difficult to carry out in practice, and they are subject to wide variation in estimates because of what may seem to be minor differences in assumptions. Severe osteoarthritis tends to be a disease of the elderly. In consequence, even an excellent functional result from joint replacement will not offset the costs of the procedure since the patient, usually past retirement age, would not re-enter the labor force regardless of treatment outcome.

Quality-of-Life Benefits

Previous chapters have emphasized the importance of enhanced quality of life as the valued outcome of surgical treatment. Joint replacement is an example of a costly intervention whose purpose is not to prolong life but rather to relieve pain and restore function, thus improving quality of life. It reminds us that although cost-effectiveness calculations may give us valuable information for policy analyses, there is a group of treatable conditions for which interventions of undeniable benefit exist but for which successful treatment will never result in recouping the original financial investment. As with other, similar interventions, the societal motivation for offering joint replacement depends more on an appreciation of the suffering experienced by a person in pain than the hope to balance all accounts.

Health-related quality of life, which concerns the capacity for self-care, freedom from pain and physical limitations, and general well-being, has become a major focus in the treatment of chronic disease. Researchers have documented improvements in patients' health-related quality of life following total joint replacement for arthritis. Krugluger and colleagues [14] evaluated the effect of total knee replacement on 340 patients averaging 68 years of age. On average, before joint replacement the patients had severe pain while attempting to walk, noted pain at rest, and disturbed sleep. At followups averaging 6 years after replacement, there was a clinically significant reduction in patients' pain levels. Similarly, before their knee replacements, 42 percent of patients had mean subjective disability scores greater than 6 on a scale of 0 to 8 (0 indicates no subjective disability; 8 indicates total dependency). At followup, these subjective disability scores showed improvement.

Hip replacement also has a beneficial effect on patients' self-image and ability to carry out activities of daily life, as well as on health perception as measured by a modified version of the Arthritis Impact Measurement Scale. In a group of 46 hip arthroplasty patients, 96 percent reported a positive change in their ability to participate in activities of daily life.

Collectively, these studies and others [6, 14] demonstrate a variety of approaches to the measurement of health-related quality of life and document the dramatic improvements among patients who undergo joint replacement.

Editors' Note

The desired outcome of surgical replacement of osteoarthritic knee or hip joints is relief of pain and improved mobility, both of which contribute to an improved quality of life. This improvement is traded against the small but finite risk to the patient of perioperative death or other complication. The financial cost of the operative procedures is roughly equivalent to that of open-heart surgery. In general, because of their ages, the successfully treated patients will not re-enter the work force. Their rehabilitation, therefore, is largely of individual rather than societal benefit. As more medical treatments come to be directed at improved quality of life rather than enhanced economic performance or survival, issues of equity, particularly intergenerational equity, will take on greater prominence.

PART H

Unanticipated Effects
of Treatment

In earlier sections of this book we have presented the idea of monitoring the health status of the population for the purpose of determining the needs of the population—for eyeglasses, dental care, immunization, or antihypertensive treatment. Another important purpose of monitoring is the early detection of unanticipated consequences of a treatment, either good or bad. The case studies reported here, regarding the treatment of peptic ulcer and the use of oral contraceptives, illustrate the need for this kind of monitoring.

About 10 percent of people are afflicted with peptic ulcer, a painful gastric disease with complications including hemorrhage and death, at some point in their lifetime. New developments in equipment—treatment through endoscopy—and drugs for treating ulcers have drastically reduced the impact of the disease. When good ideas developed from findings of basic science have produced new methods of diagnosis and treatment, however, the tendency has been to implement the new technologies and proclaim the seeming clinical successes without careful evaluation. As in the case of the milk-and-cream diet, for example, the innovation may not only not cure the ulcer, it may have unintended side effects that damage health in other ways (in this case, by promoting coronary artery disease). Only through continuing assessment can these problems be discovered.

We are all too familiar with stories about the unintended side effects of drugs. All therapeutic drugs have the potential to trigger late, adverse reactions. Most occur only rarely but may still be life-threatening. Because there is strong economic and humanitarian pressure to release new drugs for routine use as soon as possible, these late, adverse effects may be unknown prior to marketing of the drug. The need to protect patients dictates that their caregivers continue to look for adverse effects of therapeutic drugs, even though the drugs have officially been declared safe and effective by the Food and Drug Administration and approved for general use. This continued search for unexpected adverse, or sometimes beneficial, effects of approved drugs is referred to as post-marketing surveillance. Using oral contraceptive medications as an example, Chapter 15 illustrates a common and difficult problem in the evaluation of new medical treatments.

14

Peptic Ulcer

THOMAS C. CHALMERS

Background

Old as mankind, the disease called peptic ulcer can last for years, with attacks occurring once or twice a year, usually in the spring or fall. At least 10 percent of people have a peptic ulcer sometime in their lifetime. The abdominal pain is so regular and consistent that the patient can make the diagnosis better than anyone else. Not many diseases are the butt of so many jokes ("That job could give you ulcers," or "My ulcer tells . . ."). Because it can reoccur so quickly, some people repeatedly afflicted with it consider it an old friend. Yet the complications, obstruction, perforation, and hemorrhage that may ensue can be fatal. Ten percent of people with a peptic ulcer have a "massive" gastrointestinal hemorrhage, and 10 percent of them die from the bleeding or its therapy.

Probably the most intriguing aspect of peptic ulcer is its demonstration that basic biomedical research can pay off by sharply diminishing the suffering of patients prone to the disease. The ability of physicians to diagnose and treat the disease is directly the result of years of research carried out in animals and in normal and diseased people. Although the exact cause of peptic ulcer is still to be completely documented and the best modes of prevention are still to be established with certainty, the progress made in diagnosing and treating the disease in the last fifty years is one of the most remarkable accomplishments in the history of medicine.

Diagnosis

Stomach ulcers, a misnomer because the disease occurs most often in the duodenum, the organ just beyond the stomach in the alimentary canal, are relatively easy to diagnose. The typical clinical picture is familiar to most students of medicine. The pain is characteristically in the upper abdomen, and because it is associated with free acid in the stomach it comes on 2 to 3 hours after meals and is relieved, when it is not out of control, by food and antacid drugs. Patients quickly discover this themselves. The pain wakes people up at night, yet it never occurs before breakfast. It can be as regular as clockwork. Although the disease is thought to be related to stress, air traffic controllers have no greater incidence than others. In susceptible people the pain related to stress usually does not start during the stressful period before a vacation but rather after the start of vacation. That is when peptic ulcer pain hurts the most.

Medical students are taught that unless a patient with chronic recurrent upper abdominal pain has the following features, the pain is probably not due to a peptic ulcer: localized pain that comes on 2 to 4 hours after a meal, yet never before breakfast; prompt response to food or antacids; local tenderness in the upper abdomen; and regular periodic attacks, once or twice a year, often in the spring and fall. In those who still smoke the ulcer is much harder to heal.

For fifty years the diagnosis has been confirmed with relative accuracy by upper gastrointestinal x-rays. The patient swallows a liquid concoction containing the harmless element barium, which is opaque to x-rays and thus forms a silhouette of the stomach. The skilled radiologist can then outline the ulcer.

Real further progress in diagnosis was not made until one of the most remarkable technologies of modern medicine came along: fiber-optic endoscopy. Thirty-five years ago Dr. Basil Hirschowitz discovered that light transmitted along tiny flexible fibers of glass could transmit images with extreme clarity [1]. Before that, endoscopes were available to peer into the stomach, rectum, or other body orifices, but they were large and rigid, no fun to have poked into you. Fiber-optic scopes for examining every detail of the stomach or duodenum are relatively easy to swallow, and they can be used to take a piece of tissue for examination under a microscope. Engineering ingenuity and industry have combined to make fiber-optic endoscopes exquisite instruments for diagnosis and treatment. Through the endoscope, benign ulcers can usually be distinguished from malignant ones, and healing of the former can be measured with accuracy, an important step in the documentation of effective therapies.

The major advantages of fiber-optic endoscopy have been repeatedly demonstrated by reports in the medical literature. Although these reports have suffered from deficiencies only recently outlined, as investigators delineate the requirements of a scientific diagnostic evaluation, there has been a slow but probably valid "clinical" demonstration of diagnostic efficacy. The advantages of endoscopy over clinical history, physical examination, and "barium swallow" are as follows:

1. Actually viewing an ulcer allows a gastroenterologist to determine with reasonable accuracy whether it is benign or malignant, whether it is actively bleeding from an exposed blood vessel, and whether or not it has company in the form of other ulcers or diffuse inflammation of the internal lining of the stomach. Furthermore, its size is an indication of how long it will take to heal.
2. Repeated endoscopic examination allows the physician to determine with greater accuracy than by history taking the healing of an ulcer. Pain may disappear long before healing, or it may persist after healing has been demonstrated by endoscopy.
3. Small, asymptomatic ulcers that might be missed by a barium x-ray may be demonstrated by endoscopy.
4. Valuable procedures such as tissue biopsies and localized treatments can be carried out through the endoscope.

The disadvantages of upper gastrointestinal endoscopy are:

1. Accidental perforation of the esophagus or stomach may occur, although questionnaire surveys indicate that it happens in fewer than one in a thousand endoscopies.
2. It may take years of "scoping" patients before the operator is skilled enough at passing and using the scope in a sufficient variety and number of patients. Any procedure in medicine that is dependent on human observation has an observer error rate that is diminished but not eliminated by experience, as may be demonstrated by having two observers make an endoscopic diagnosis without prior data on the patient and without knowing what the other found. Clinically important differences may occur between 5 and 20 percent of the time.
3. Endoscopy is a time-consuming procedure that takes gastroenterologists away from other valuable procedures, such as skillfully taking a patient's history.
4. The cost can be high, because of the need to purchase constantly

updated instruments and because of the skill required from the personnel, both the operators and their assistants. A dedicated room is also required.

5. If endoscopy is not performed with discretion and skill, the health care costs potentially saved by more accurate diagnosis can be negated by the increased costs of the procedure.

As is so often the case in clinical medicine, an accurate and unbiased comparison of the diagnostic accuracy of endoscopy and barium x-ray has not yet been reported. There are many papers comparing them, but the conclusions are more associated with the clinical discipline of the author than with an unbiased evaluation of the data. Radiologists publish papers documenting the relative efficacy of radiology [2], and endoscopists make the same claim for endoscopy. At the present time, clinical experience seems to favor endoscopy, except under special circumstances.

Soon after the widespread use of endoscopy began, but before treatment with endoscopy was introduced, it was hypothesized that the more accurate diagnosis of the site and severity of bleeding from the upper gastrointestinal tract should obviously lead to the savings of lives. Five gastroenterologists conducted clinical trials in which patients were randomly assigned to early endoscopy or to a regimen that excluded endoscopy unless a special indication arose. There was agreement about the outcome among all five studies. In each case the death rate in hospital was slightly increased with endoscopy, and pooling of the data revealed little chance that the employment of early endoscopy for *diagnostic* purposes could reduce the hospital death rate. As discussed below under "Treatment," the later introduction of the ability to treat the bleeding ulcer successfully through the scope dramatically changed the usefulness of endoscopy. Nowadays every patient presenting with upper gastrointestinal hemorrhage should be scoped immediately, and if an ulcer is found it should be treated. The important change in the management of ulcers is discussed in detail below.

Treatment

Until about 1983, the only effective treatments for bleeding ulcers were blood transfusions, diet, drugs, and abdominal surgery. The last three were based on the "no acid, no ulcer!" hypothesis. Keep something in the stomach and the acid would not be able to eat away at the tissues unprotected by the gastric or duodenal "mucosa." In fact, the remarkable ability of that mucosa to resist the pepsin that digests ordinary protein in an acid medium has been the subject of intensive basic research, as part of the effort to understand peptic ulcers so they can be better prevented and treated.

Partial appreciation of the cause of peptic ulcers resulted in classic examples of the vastly misguided treatment of patients that can result from the application of scientific knowledge without adequate clinical trials designed to determine efficacy and toxicity. Protecting and healing the gastric mucosa were approached with one or more of three ways to neutralize the offending digestive acids: diet, acid-neutralizing drugs, and surgical removal of the ulcer or acid-secreting cells. Undertaking clinical trials of treatments based on basic science knowledge is not what I am criticizing in this chapter. Rather, I fault the subsequent step: when clinicians first tried their ideas in sick patients, they abandoned the principles of the scientific method that had been employed in the basic research. Faced with a relentlessly progressing and distressing disease, they tried each

The Accidental Volunteer

The early studies of the effects of food and stress on the physiology of the stomach lining provide a classic example of the synergy of curiosity on the one side and opportunity in the form of a "natural experiment" on the other. William Beaumont, a U.S. Army surgeon stationed at Fort Mackinac, attended a *voyageur* named Alexis St. Martin who had accidentally been hit by a shotgun blast to his left side from a distance of about three feet. St. Martin did survive the wound under Beaumont's care, but it healed in a way that left a persistent and sizable opening between the inside of his stomach and the outside world.

Recognizing the opportunity, Beaumont undertook a series of experiments on the now-healed St. Martin in which he observed the lining of the stomach and the changes in its contents in the course of feeding, fasting, and emotion. The experiments continued intermittently over the next eight years. Upon publication of the results in 1834, Beaumont's work was immediately recognized by physicians and physiologists as having landmark importance. Beaumont ultimately settled into an active practice in St. Louis; St. Martin returned to a hardscrabble farm in his native Canada.

new idea as it came along, and if happy success occurred with more patients than they might have expected, they published their results. As others confirmed the occasional superiority of their treatment over past methods, they began to bask in the glory.

Undoubtedly the scientific need for adequate controls was appreciated, but establishing control groups would require withholding treatment for an observational period or assigning patients by chance to the standard therapy. That course seemed improper to some investigators, in view of the fact that the patient had been sent to them for help and they *believed* that their new idea was better than any other treatment available. All of the treatments no longer in vogue probably reached popularity via this kind of reasoning: an idea emerging from basic scientific research, a con-secutive series of patients with apparently good outcomes reported at medical meetings and in the medical literature, agreement and celebration at the meetings and on the editorial pages, and further reports of success. Adverse outcomes were seldom reported, unless the writer had time to spare or an alternative innovation to propose. Many of the once-popular medical and surgical treatments were abandoned later, but only after thousands of patients were treated suboptimally who might not have been had they been randomly assigned to a control group in a scientific study.

In 1915 Sippy [3] first reported that ulcers could be cured if the patient would drink a mixture of milk and cream every two hours, night and day, and take antacids in between. Others vigorously advocated a bland diet, often soft food only, and these rapidly became the widely accepted norms for peptic ulcer treatment. It was years before several randomized control trials (RCTs) showed that although frequent ingestion of food might be important, the content of the diet mattered not. Furthermore, information began to emerge in the cardiovascular community, apparently not appre-ciated by the majority of gastroenterologists, that excessive cream in the diet could cause fatal coronary artery disease. So the improperly evaluated treatment was not only unnecessary but was also potentially harmful. If Sippy had known enough to assign volunteering patients at random to his liquid diet or a normal diet, he would have discovered early that the milk-and-cream diet was unnecessary. Instead, it was years before the proper trials were done, and years after that some physicians were still ordering a Sippy diet for patients with duodenal ulcers [4]. Such is the slow pace of medicine when physicians are not trained to perform proper clinical trials soon after an innovation is introduced or do not believe the results when the trials have been performed.

Another example of the need for proper early clinical trials has to do with surgical intervention for chronic or recurrent peptic ulcer. The idea of removing parts or most of the stomach quickly became popular because patients who survived the operations had fewer relapses of their ulcers. They often suffered from complications of surgery, however, and literally thousands of modifications of the original gastrectomy operation have appeared in the surgical literature. Except for some multi-treatment randomized control trials carried out by the cooperative studies program of the Veterans Administration, practically none of the attempts to modify the classical gastrectomy operation were evaluated by proper control trials.

One of these modifications gained popularity thirty years ago, at a time when people had begun to appreciate that selecting suitable patients at random was both an ethical and rapid way to demonstrate relative efficacy. The original uncontrolled trials of a new surgical approach, vagotomy, or cutting the vagus nerves that stimulate acid secretion, revealed that ulcer symptoms could be relieved by an operation that was much simpler than removing more and more of the stomach, but again the side effects were annoying. Interruption of the other functions of the vagus nerve were causing trouble. This time, with some exceptions, the modifications selected to overcome these difficulties were properly explored. Patients receiving various specialized vagotomy operations, involving the laborious dissection primarily of those fibers in the vagus that control acid secretion, were compared with randomly selected patients receiving the standard truncal vagotomy.

Around this time a respected surgeon, Owen Wangensteen, Chairman of the Department of Surgery at the University of Minnesota, sought a nonsurgical approach to curing peptic ulcer. He demonstrated in dogs that freezing the lining of the stomach could permanently lower the secretion of acid. Selected patients with ulcers resistant to medical treatment (frequent ingestion of a soft or bland diet and antacid drugs) received a new treatment: a balloon at the end of a two-channel tube was placed in their stomachs, and a freezing solution was circulated inside the balloon until it was estimated that the acid-secreting cells had been permanently damaged. Many papers in the surgical literature reported dramatic cures in uncontrolled trials carried out in patients with recurrent and chronic peptic ulcer. The result was that almost every hospital purchased and began to use the apparatus for "freezing" the stomach. News of life-threatening complications and failures to cure at the same rate as reported by the innovator began to appear in the medical literature. Doubts began to arise as to whether patients were better off being treated with this procedure, surgery, or conservative medical therapy. Fortunately, several gastroenterologists undertook randomized control trials comparing freezing with standard therapy. Some were small trials and some were large, cooperative studies. None revealed a significant benefit from freezing, and pooling the small trials suggested that if there was any benefit it was very small.

Here, it is important to interrupt in order to review the benefits of meta-analysis, a relatively new statistical technique that facilitates much more rapid and effective analysis of randomized control trials of new and old therapies and evaluation of diagnostic interventions. Very often trials of therapeutic and diagnostic interventions have so few patients that valid conclusions may not be made about whether the results warrant adoption of the therapeutic intervention or whether they are easily explained by the play of chance. That decision leans on statistical analyses to tell us how far chance fluctuations go toward explaining the departure of the data from displaying equality of performance of the interventions being tested. Even when two treatments are equally effective, when their performance is compared in a small number of patients one of the treatments will usually appear to perform better. We need to observe a big enough difference to be persuaded that one treatment is preferable, or employ a big enough sample to tell us that whatever difference may exist is too small for clinical concern.

The degree of difference is often expressed as a p value, defined as the probability of observing at least as big a difference as the one obtained if the two treatments were actually equal in performance. Often the criterion of a p value being less than 0.05 is taken as a cue that the observed difference is not readily explainable by chance fluctuations. In statistical jargon, such small p values show "statistical significance of the difference in performance at the 5 percent level." One hopes that such a cue is pointing toward better performance by one of the treatments, but another possibility is that some bias in the study is creating the difference.

A small study is not likely to achieve statistical significance at the 5 percent level or less, whether or not one of the therapies is more effective. Therefore, a finding of nonsignificance from a small study still leaves the possibility that there is a clinically important difference in performance between the treatments. Combining several well-designed studies that ask the same questions and use the same endpoints can increase the effective sample size and increase the probability that an actual performance difference will be detected by the *p* value method. The methods used for such quantitative combining are sometimes called "meta-analyses," sometimes "overviews." Meta-analysis of a number of small trials thus allows conclusions to be drawn that are not possible on the basis of the individual studies alone. Although *p* values are used to announce the statistical significance of the effect of treatment, the size of the effect is of primary importance—the reduction in death rate or the increased percentage of cures.

In the case of vagotomy for peptic ulcer, the individual trials revealed a trend toward fewer complications and an increased ulcer relapse rate with the newer operation [5]. When these results were combined in meta-analyses, it was apparent that the differences were highly statistically significant, facilitating the decision about which operation was preferable. A higher ulcer relapse rate was acceptable because other ulcer treatments could be tried in the patients whose treatment failed. A higher rate of complications of vagotomy was not acceptable, because not much could be done about the distressing complications of vagotomy.

In the case of gastric freezing, there was also a trend toward decreased relapses of the ulcers when the randomized control trials (RCTs) were combined, but the trend was of small magnitude and clinically less impressive than the side effects of freezing. So the freezing apparatuses were relegated to the storerooms of the hospitals that had spent valuable resources to purchase them.

Meanwhile, basic pharmacologic research has made all surgery for peptic ulcer much less needed. It had been known for half a century that a substance called histamine, the same substance known to mediate allergic reactions, was involved in the response of gastric mucosal cells to acid-secreting stimuli. But drugs that block allergic reactions and relieve the symptoms of people with hayfever, histamine-1 blockers, now sold over the counter, have little or no effect on acid secretion. However, a British pharmacologist, Sir James Whyte Black, discovered a class of drugs, called histamine-2 blockers, that dramatically inhibit the secretion of gastric acid, with minimal side effects. Sales of the first of these agents, cimetidine, skyrocketed, because it was used not only to treat and prevent peptic ulcer but also to relieve much more common and benign forms of indigestion. In contrast to earlier drugs for peptic ulcer, there have been over a thousand RCTs evaluating histamine-2 blockers in patients with peptic ulcers and related diseases, as well as many meta-analyses of those trials.

The latest saga in the development of better methods of treating and preventing recurrent peptic ulcer emerges from research on a bacterium that has been known by many names, the present one being *Helicobacter pylori*. The association of the bacterium with peptic ulcer has been known for years. Yet all acknowledged that it was unclear whether the growth of the bacterium was the result of or the cause of recurrent peptic ulcer. Several RCTs of antibiotic therapy suggested that the bacterium might play a causative role, and that idea has been confirmed by a large-scale RCT [6]. Although the histamine-2 blockers are moderately successful in preventing recurrent ulcers, combination with antibiotic treatment may prove to be highly effective. We eagerly await meta-analyses of the many antibacterial trials in patients with peptic ulcer to determine the true usefulness of this approach. Dramatic as the histamine-2 blockers have been in healing acute ulcers, their record in prevention of recurrences has been spotty (another reason for more meta-analyses of the many trials now being carried out).

Bleeding Peptic Ulcer

The dramatic history of this complication of peptic ulcer is treated as a separate section of this chapter because it illustrates so well the improper and proper evaluations of technological advances. Over 150 papers have been found in the medical literature that report both the frequency of emergency surgical intervention and the rate of death in hospital of patients with peptic ulcers admitted with signs of hemorrhage. In the last half-century, the rate of "rescue" by surgery has increased from under 5 to over 70 percent of the patients in each individual report. Although the hospital death rates vary from 0 to over 20 percent, depending on the number of patients and severity of the illness in each report, the average death rate has stayed at 10 percent throughout this period of increasing surgical intervention. Four randomized control trials comparing the mortality outcome of early emergency surgical intervention with that of conservative therapy and surgery only when continued bleeding demands it have been reported. The first three showed "no difference" in outcome, but they were small enough to have missed a clinically important benefit or harm. One showed a significant reduction in mortality with early surgery. All four of the randomized control trials had the unavoidable defect that too many patients assigned to emergency surgery never received it, and many assigned to medical care had emergency surgery because of continued bleeding. It is still unclear whether a policy of early surgical intervention would save some patients who might die without it. The advent of successful endoscopic treatment probably makes the question moot.

Endoscopic treatment of bleeding peptic ulcers is a wonderful example of how lives can be saved, unnecessary surgery prevented, and patient discomfort sharply reduced by the prompt administration of randomized control trials to evaluate the efficacy of a new technology. It is also a beautiful demonstration of the value of starting randomized control trials early and performing meta-analyses of all the published trials early. Originally it was thought that prompt endoscopy might reduce mortality by facilitating an early accurate diagnosis. Pooling of the five published trials comparing mortality in patients assigned at random either to early diagnostic endoscopy or conventional treatment revealed that hospital mortality was if anything increased by using diagnostic endoscopy when no effective therapy was available. Then a number of gastroenterologists got the idea that treating the bleeding vessel, or the ulcer from which the bleeding seemed to have come, with heat, an electric current, a laser, or injection of a tissue-damaging fluid might stop the bleeding, reduce the need for emergency surgery, and even reduce hospital mortality. To their everlasting credit, the endoscopists recognized that an RCT was the most effective and ethical way to establish as rapidly as possible the efficacy or dangers of the new treatment. Within a few years after treatment of the first patient, RCTs began to be reported. Most RCTs were too small to demonstrate efficacy in themselves. The collection of completed RCTs, properly pooled using meta-analysis, could have demonstrated by 1982 that endoscopic treatment was effective. The new treatment halved the rates of continued or recurrent bleeding, halved the need for emergency surgical intervention, and reduced the hospital death rate by 30 percent. In fact, it is the first treatment ever to be shown conclusively to lower the hospital death rate from bleeding peptic ulcer. It is a clear-cut triumph for the engineers who developed the therapeutic flexible fiber-optic endoscope, for the gastroenterologists who thought of the idea and employed early RCTs to evaluate efficacy of the treatment, and for the meta-analysts who put together the published RCTs for the first demonstration that the death rate from bleeding peptic ulcer could be reduced.

This result is an excellent example of the fact that performing meta-analyses at regular intervals can establish efficacy early in the development of a new technology. Not long after the first trial, the hospital death rate was shown to be reduced from 10 to 7 percent, a 30 percent reduction, the first documented improvement in survival of patients with bleeding peptic ulcer in fifty years. Cumulative meta-analysis, the process of repeating meta-analyses of all suitable trials each time a new trial is reported, promises to be a major innovation in health care. It should greatly shorten the time now lost between the moment of general agreement to adopt an effective therapy and the actual discarding of an ineffective one previously in use. Both types of delay are serious impediments to holding down the costs of medical care.

Cumulative meta-analysis has its critics, and there are details still to be worked out. The mere attainment of statistical significance or failure to achieve it does not mean that an innovative therapy should be universally adopted or rejected. There are other issues for health policy authorities to consider—side effects, other available treatments, relative cost and availability—but no rational decisions should be made without referral to reliable data, and carrying out cumulatively updated meta-analyses of well-done randomized control trials is the best way to supply those data.

In summary, peptic ulcer is a common disease of mankind that is gradually being conquered by the application of the scientific method in the form of randomized control trials to the practice of medicine. That is the reason for reviewing the history of peptic ulcer diagnosis, treatment, and prevention in detail. It is a good model for demonstrating proper and improper ways to adopt or reject technical innovations designed to help people with a specific disease.

Editors' Note

By following the historical development of diagnosis and treatment of peptic ulcer, this chapter illustrates the contributions of basic medical science and, at the same time, the need for randomized control trials before dissemination of science-based clinical treatments. Basic science offers good suggestions for possible treatments, but unless the resulting innovations are tested carefully at the time of their introduction, the new treatments cannot be assumed to be effective. The examples here of the Sippy diet, of gastric freezing, and of endoscopy for diagnosis alone (rather than endoscopic treatment) all show the hazards of disseminating procedures without benefit of rigorous assessment.

The urgency of treatment presses the clinician to use new treatments and believe in their effectiveness even without comparative randomized trials. Yet when treatments have not been adequately tested, patients have often been put to the trouble and expense of treatments that have turned out to be ineffective or even harmful. A basic problem for clinicians that has never been resolved is how certain one can ethically be without empirical evidence favoring a treatment. The problem cannot be entirely resolved, because there will never be enough data to assure the effectiveness of a given treatment for a specific patient, and clinicians always need to interpolate between the evidence from research and the application for the patient at hand. This chapter illustrates that thoroughgoing assessment of innovations, including meta-analytic studies of the sort reviewed here, is required to provide the research evidence on which to base these clinical decisions.

15

Oral Contraceptives: Post-Marketing Surveillance and Rare, Late Complications of Drugs

HOWARD S. FRAZIER AND GRAHAM A. COLDITZ

Background

Oral contraceptive drugs have stimulated more clinical studies of more women by more investigators than any other family of medicines in history. Their popularity among women has been just as remarkable. In the group of women born after 1945, some 80 percent had used the drugs before they reached the age of 35. Given this widespread use and the extent of study of these medicines, it may seem unlikely that anything useful remains to be said about oral contraceptives. Although the drugs are immensely successful in fostering reproductive choice, their use reminds us of a series of crucial questions that required answers early in the development of oral contraceptives, questions that will often be asked in the future about novel and widely used medical technologies.

The most common objective for the use of oral contraceptives is the safe, reliable, convenient, and reversible control of fertility. We take as a given that the drugs are very effective in reducing the risk of unwanted pregnancy—they are highly effective contraceptives. Their success in achieving this goal will insure their use by large numbers of healthy women over long periods of time to prevent an outcome, pregnancy, that imposes a relatively low risk of death on the mother. This combination of wide use and low risk of harm to a woman who does become pregnant sets stringent conditions for our assessment of oral contraceptives.

The purpose of this chapter is, first, to consider what evidence should be gathered to evaluate oral contraceptives for wide use by women. Our second goal is to identify some unanticipated risks and benefits of the use of oral contraceptives, and to describe some of the methodologies that have been developed to detect uncommon events that may be caused by the treatment. Finally and more broadly, we ask whether our present approach to evaluating widely disseminated medical technologies is adequate to guide their use.

The Efficacy and Risks of Oral Contraceptives

In the three decades since their introduction, the active ingredients of the oral contraceptives have undergone substantial change. The types in widest use in the United States in 1993 contain very low doses of derivatives of the female sex hormones estrogen and progesterone, compared with the levels of these hormones in the pills first introduced. We accept the evidence, not reviewed here, that the drugs are highly effective agents for the prevention of pregnancy—pregnancy rates per 1,000 woman-years of use as low as 1 to 10 are standard [1].

Knowing that efficacy is high is not very informative without estimates of the risks of chronic use of the drugs. We compare this risk with that of maternal death associated with pregnancy. In Table 15-1, modified from Tietze [2], the risk of maternal death per 100,000 pregnancies ending in a live birth is shown for each five-year interval of women's peak reproductive years. Note that in the column headed "Pregnancy and childbirth" the risk of death for the mother goes through a minimum in the 20–24-year age group and then rises steadily with age to a value of risk of death in the 40–44-year age group approximately seven times the minimum.

Now we ask whether this age-related risk of maternal death from unwanted pregnancy and delivery is more or less than the risk of death each year, for equivalent age groups, experienced by a woman who takes the oral contraceptive and prevents a pregnancy. In short, setting aside the important question of an individual's preference about fertility control, is it riskier to go through a pregnancy or to prevent the pregnancy by taking oral contraceptives for a year?

To answer this question, we compare in Table 15-1 the figures in the columns headed "Pregnancy and childbirth" and "Oral contraceptive use with no tobacco." (We will return shortly to the significance of specifying no tobacco use.) The table shows that for each age group, the risk of maternal death in the course of a pregnancy is roughly ten times the risk to a woman of taking an oral contraceptive that will almost certainly

Table 15-1. Mortality rates in women from pregnancy and childbirth and from use of oral contraceptives.

Age group	Mortality per 100,000 live births or users per year		
	Pregnancy and childbirth	Oral contraceptive use with—	
		No tobacco	Tobacco
15–19	11.1	1.2	1.4
20–24	10.0	1.2	1.4
25–29	12.5	1.2	1.4
30–34	24.9	1.8	10.4
35–39	44.0	3.9	12.8
40–44	71.4	6.6	58.4

Source: Based on data used with the permission of The Alan Guttmacher Institute from Christopher Tietze, "New Estimates of Mortality Associated with Fertility Control," *Family Planning Perspectives,* vol. 9, no. 2, March/April 1977.

prevent a pregnancy. Note that these facts describe only the risks of pregnancy and delivery and the risk of a year's use of the medicine. No comparison with other methods of fertility control is intended. We began by asking what kinds of additional information we should seek in evaluating the technology of oral contraceptives. The fact that these medications are female sex hormones or hormone analogues immediately suggests that in fulfilling our first objective of evaluating the drugs for wide use, we should monitor effects, developing in the short term, on organs related to reproduction: uterus, uterine cervix, breast, and ovary. As will become obvious, this approach has serious limitations.

Our second objective is to identify unanticipated effects of the use of the oral contraceptives. The long latent period that elapses before the effects of some drugs are expressed, and the seriousness of the effects that can develop after the latent period, is well documented. The evaluation of the safety and efficacy of new drugs required by the Food and Drug Administration generally works well in detecting acute adverse effects of the types already familiar to investigators. Systems for the detection of late effects involving novel complications, however, are not as well developed. One reason is the difficulty in designing a detection system when we don't know precisely what we are trying to detect. Two examples illustrate the point.

A young woman was being treated for a gynecologic disorder with female sex hormones. In the course of her treatment, she suffered from a pulmonary embolism, a blood clot that moved from the veins of her lower body to her lungs, a potentially lethal event. Her physician speculated that the hormonal treatment may have increased her susceptibility to intravascular clotting and embolism, although this connection had not previously been documented. The case and the speculation were reported in 1961 and other investigations, focused now by a specific, testable hypothesis, soon confirmed that the hormonal treatment did increase the risk of pulmonary embolism. On the inspiration of this single physician hinged the discovery of a significant, unanticipated side effect; it was not detected by any system designed routinely to monitor and identify adverse effects of medications.

Another example of the discovery of an unanticipated consequence of oral contraceptive use is the real but unexplained interaction between tobacco use, oral contraceptives, and intravascular clotting and embolism in young women. The relevant comparison is found in the two righthand columns of Table 15-1, which show the mortality observed per 100,000 oral contraceptive user-years as a function of age and smoking status. Among oral contraceptive users in the age groups of 30 and above, tobacco use greatly increased the age-dependent risk of death in these women.

Consequences of oral contraceptive use that are not directly measured by fertility control may take decades to become apparent, and therefore any interpretation of the nonreproductive effects of the changes in oral contraceptive composition over time must be conservative. That said, the doses of the hormones in current contraceptive pills are substantially lower than the levels in earlier formulations. For that reason, we expect that nonreproductive consequences noted in the women on current dose levels will be less likely or less profound than the effects in the original cohorts of contraceptive users.

Detecting Rare, Late Outcomes of Oral Contraceptive Use

We have mentioned that one strategy for monitoring for unanticipated events related to oral contraceptive use is to look for effects on organs and tissues related to reproduction. Although a reasonable, if narrow, approach, this one will not regularly lead us to outcomes that we cannot, in advance, connect with the causal event, in this case the use of oral contraceptives.

The epidemiologist tries to discover causal connections between events.

When the events of interest are relatively common—for example, the occurrence of measles in children who have or have not been immunized—it usually is easy to design and carry out an experimental clinical trial. Because the events are common, enough of them can be observed among randomly allocated experimental and control groups so that even small differences between them attain statistical significance. When the events of interest are uncommon, it may be impossible to gather enough observations to set up a controlled trial. Under these circumstances, the investigator may have to give up the strongest study design and pursue the weaker, more bias-prone, alternative approaches, such as a cohort study, case-control study, or series of cases (see Chapter 2).

Ordinarily, we expect that the late, rare consequences of oral contraceptive use inevitably will be adverse. In order to emphasize the importance to adequate surveillance of maintaining an open mind about the characteristics of late, rare effects, we cite two counterexamples.

Cancer of the ovary is common but difficult to diagnose at an early stage; five-year survival rates for women diagnosed with ovarian cancer are, on average, less than 20 percent. These grim characteristics point up the importance of any increase in prevalence of the disease due to oral contraceptives, as well as the desirability of discovering ways to reduce the risk. Both case-control and cohort studies have been used to examine what association there may be between ovarian cancer and oral contraceptives. They show that use of the drugs for as short an interval as five years reduced the risk of subsequent ovarian cancer to 50 percent or less of the risk to non-users. Furthermore, the protective effect persists for at least fifteen years [1].

Prior use of oral contraceptives has a similar beneficial effect on the risk of cancer of the endometrium, the lining of the uterus. As was the case with ovarian cancer, the beneficial effect of prior oral contraceptive use on the incidence of endometrial cancer was apparent for at least 15 years after use [1].

By contrast, prior use of the oral contraceptives is associated with an increase in cancer of the liver. An increase in the rate of heart attacks in current users of oral contraceptives was noted early in the history of hormonal contraception. In the early 1990s, research results tend, however, to show no increase in risk of cardiovascular disease.

These examples indicate the complexity of the problem of detecting and quantifying some of the effects of therapeutic drugs: the effects may be rare and widely separated in time from the original use of the drug, they need have no predictable relationship to the major effects of the drug, and they may be either harmful or beneficial. These characteristics impose a set of stringent demands on any surveillance system.

Post-Marketing Surveillance

Although the phrase "post-marketing surveillance" (PMS) could be applied to any technology that has been approved by some licensing body for use in the health sector, it has come to refer mainly to the monitoring of new drugs after their release to the medical market. As we have noted earlier, the Food and Drug Administration's pre-marketing requirements for new drugs are directed primarily at the determination of efficacy and the detection of acute, familiar, adverse reactions. After approval for safety and efficacy by the FDA and the release of the drug to the market, particularly if the drug is likely to be as widely used as oral contraceptives, the evaluation enlarges to include discovery of rare, late outcomes of its use. In addition, with the passage of time, improved knowledge may suggest further avenues for exploration.

Although the need for post-marketing surveillance is widely acknowledged among health professionals, as yet we have not progressed beyond a voluntary reporting system for events that are recognized as adverse drug reactions by the reporting health worker. Not unexpectedly for a system that leaves the initiative entirely in the hands of the health worker, reporting rates are low. An equally serious disadvantage is that, because the target is adverse drug reactions, the system tends to detect the known effects and overlook adverse events that are novel and that *may* be drug-related.

There is hope of doing better. First, the increase in power and decline in price of small computers brings in reach the recording of all, or a sample of all, prescriptions for a set of new drugs, the name and address of the prescribing physician, and a patient identifier that may be held in confidence. A system for post-marketing surveillance has been developed and tried in Great Britain as an independent charitable trust under the direction of its originator, Professor W. H. W. Inman of the University of Southampton [3]. The system, known as prescription-event monitoring, has a number of important features. First, it monitors *events* (any untoward happening occurring to a patient) in identified patients whose prescriptions and physicians are matters of record within the system. It does not attempt to monitor adverse drug reactions, because the identification of adverse reactions may be biased. Recognition that a particular event is related to a particular medication is made on the basis of the pattern of association of event and drug across very large numbers of patients and exposures to the drug. Second, the surveillance system contacts the physician after an appropriate period of time to enquire about the possible occurrence of events in the course of the patient of interest, the patient having been identified on the basis of a prescription. Third, the system has the capacity to monitor almost every patient who receives a newly introduced medication in a defined population. Fourth, up to approximately 20 drugs can be studied at a given time. The usual cohort for a drug is about 20,000 individuals. Fifth, the costs of the system seem to be adjustable according to the desired capacity.

Other countries are experimenting with other systems to accomplish similar purposes.

Conclusions

In considering systems for post-marketing surveillance, it may appear that we have strayed far from the topic of oral contraceptive drugs. The connection can easily be re-established, however. New chemical entities, and modifications of familiar ones, are being introduced into the practice of medicine at prodigious rates. Each of these drugs offers the promise of healing, sometimes in ways we do not anticipate. Each also offers the prospect of harm, sometimes remote and usually unexpected.

In order to balance benefits and risks in the interest of patients, we need detailed, quantitative information about the effects of medications, first in the short term. As a practical matter, we choose not to delay release of what seems to be a useful new drug while we study it for rare, late outcomes. The result is that we must continue to monitor the effects of new drugs long after they have been introduced into practice. As we have seen in the case of oral contraceptives, failure to establish effective post-marketing surveillance condemns us to suffer late ill effects, or to miss opportunities to reap benefits we had not anticipated.

Editors' Note

Post-marketing surveillance in the United States is accomplished by voluntary reports from individual health professionals regarding suspected adverse events, some two-thirds of which are related to drugs.

The reports may be sent either to the manufacturer or to the Food and Drug Administration. As might be expected in a voluntary system, underreporting appears to be common. In addition, since the reporter usually is reporting what is thought to be an adverse reaction to a drug, the system is biased toward detecting events that look like previously observed drug reactions, at the expense of missing unusual kinds of adverse events.

In the case of oral contraceptives, it was largely chance that led ultimately to the discovery of important adverse events, previously unrecognized as drug-related, caused by the formation of blood clots in the blood vessels of the legs, pelvis, brain, and heart of women who smoked while using oral contraceptives. The case presented in this chapter illustrates the need for a more coordinated monitoring system. It shows that counting adverse events related to the drug's antecedents, here reproductive effects, does not yield the most useful information. Detecting late, rare, and unexpected effects of such a widely used drug is the critical matter.

Other nations have developed more effective systems of post-marketing surveillance than the United States has. The British, for example, have developed a system that captures "events" happening to a patient who received a prescription for a particular drug. On a routine, systematic, and continuing basis, the patient's physician is queried about that patient's course and the occurrence of any unusual events. Unexpected associations between administration of the drug and "events" occurring in the population can be noted and subjected to additional statistical tests.

The label "drug reaction" has the connotation of a harmful result, but it need not be so. Rigorous clinical studies of women treated with oral contraceptives show that use of the drugs for periods as short as five years in the past cuts down the long-term risk of developing cancers of the ovary or uterine lining to roughly half the risk found in women who have not been treated with oral contraceptives.

The overall lesson to be learned from the history of oral contraceptives and the design of systems for post-marketing surveillance is that careful, rigorous clinical trials can identify which interventions work and which do not, and they can also discover unanticipated hazards and, sometimes, unexpected benefits.

PART I

Administrative Innovations

Our final case study involves an organizational innovation: the evolution of multidisciplinary teams of professionals for the provision of increasingly complex and successful surgical care. We ordinarily think of medical technology as a piece of equipment that is designed to accomplish a particular purpose. Yet it is just as appropriate to regard a new configuration of groups of people as a technological innovation: a team that makes possible the accomplishment of new tasks.

We recognize that many aspects of daily life, including nutrition, shelter, and societal stability, make an important positive contribution to health status. Given these "outside" factors and the complexity of current medical procedures, it is difficult to assign responsibility for improvements in outcome to particular members of a surgical team. For our purposes, it is sufficient to ask what *measurable* benefits the surgical team contributes to human health, and in what ways might the outcomes of treatment by the surgical team be improved. For that reason, Chapter 16 puts most emphasis on the overall performance of the surgical team as measured by patient outcomes of particular surgical treatments.

16

Surgery and Anesthesiology

DEBRA R. MILAMED AND JOHN HEDLEY-WHYTE

Introduction

In his autobiographical memoir, *A Twentieth Century Surgeon* [1], Dr. Claude E. Welch of the Massachusetts General Hospital cites twenty outstanding medical developments of the twentieth century that in his opinion have had more impact than all previous advances in the history of medicine:

An enormous increase in the percentage of the gross national product devoted to health care.

A dramatic change in hospital activities. Lengths of patient stays have been shortened for nearly all diseases and procedures. Relatively simple operations are now done in ambulatory facilities. Expensive machines such as equipment for computerized tomography and magnetic resonance imaging are standard equipment; many hospitals have extensive research programs. Hospital costs have escalated enormously because of these factors.

Improved methods of anesthesia and respiratory care.

Cardiac surgery.

Organ transplantation.

Expansion of pharmaceuticals and instrumentation, e.g. flexible endoscopy and laparoscopic procedures.

Several of these developments are most clearly evident in the modern practice of surgery, which the preface to *Costs, Risks, and Benefits of Surgery*

[2] has termed representative of "medical care at its greatest complexity and highest cost."

Between 20 and 25 million operations requiring general anesthesia are performed in the United States each year. It is estimated that the average operation generates $5,000 in direct costs to either the patient or the insurance carrier, bringing the total to $125 billion annually. In recent years both public and private sectors have expressed growing concern about possibly inappropriate surgical procedures adding to the increasingly high national health care expenditures. In this chapter we review some advances in modern surgical care and related factors underlying the decrease in mortality attributable to selected diseases treated by surgery during the period 1968–1988 [3]. At the same time, we recognize the impact on mortality over time of changing demographics, socioeconomic trends, and other factors beyond the scope of this chapter.

Anesthesia and the recognition of the need for infection control, which led to the development of aseptic techniques toward the close of the nineteenth century, transformed the science and practice of surgery [1]. The first public demonstration of ether anesthesia, by Doctors Warren and Morton at the Massachusetts General Hospital in 1846, has been termed the most significant single event in nineteenth-century medicine [1]. F. Treves, in his 1900 address to a British medical society [4], described the enormous impact of anesthesia on surgical practice. Before anesthesia, most operations consisted of treatment of wounds and fractures, especially those acquired on the battlefield, the removal of stones from the urinary tract (lithotomy), amputations, and the treatment of hemorrhages and fistulas. In the popular imagination, surgeons had been rough characters of low prestige, although even before the midnineteenth century some had achieved high academic positions and improved social standing [5]. The use of anesthetics enabled the surgeon to enter the abdominal cavity, while "Listerism"—the use of carbolic acid spray to control bacteria in the operating room—dramatically improved postoperative survival. In 1888 the Massachusetts General Hospital built its first abdominal surgery ward [1].

A third breakthrough, the acquisition of appropriate knowledge and technology for the transfusion of human blood, began with the basic work of K. Landsteiner in 1901 [5]. By the late 1930s many cities worldwide had blood transfusion units.

Effective infection control led to the opening of numerous new hospitals at the close of the nineteenth century, particularly those affiliated with universities and medical schools. Some of these hospitals began to operate professional training schools for nurses. Between 1880 and 1948 the number of such schools rose from 15 to over 1,500 [6].

By the turn of the century, the surgeon was becoming a specialist. William S. Halsted introduced the residency system and opened a laboratory for surgical research. As a result of a committee report issued in 1912, the American College of Surgeons was formed in 1913. The work of this committee also led to the creation of the Joint Commission on the Accreditation of Hospitals (JCAH, now JCAHO) ten years later. The introduction to the *Summary Report of the Study on Surgical Services in the United States* (SOSSUS) [6], prepared by a national committee formed by the American Surgical Association and the American College of Surgeons, points out the importance of the advances made in these areas in the period 1920–1945: the development of standards for hospitals, the certification of internships and residencies, the creation of specialty boards, and the approval of medical schools.

Changes in Mortality and Hospital Care, 1968–1988

For decades the treatment of some relatively common diseases—appendicitis, gallbladder disease (or cholecystitis) and gallstones (cholelithiasis), gastric and duodenal ulcer, hernia and intestinal obstruction, and benign hyperplasia of the prostate—has typified the "bread-and-butter" surgery of the medium-sized American hospital. We used published *Vital Statistics* data from the National Center for Health Statistics (NCHS) to study changes in mortality attributable to these causes for the years 1968, 1978, and 1988 among individuals aged 15 and over (in the case of benign prostate hyperplasia, males aged 45 and over) in the United States. These years were selected because sufficient data were available to furnish a "case study" spanning two decades [3]. We analyzed mortality data, rather than information on actual rates of operative success or failure, simply because the latter type of data has not been compiled in a uniform and usable manner over time.

Figure 16-1 illustrates a dramatic fall in the death rates from these diseases, with the steepest declines occurring during the interval 1968 to 1978 [3]. During the same period, average lengths of hospital stay reported by NCHS for patients of all ages (males aged 45 and over in the case of benign prostate hyperplasia) for whom these diseases were their primary diagnoses were also reduced (see Figure 16-2).

We reviewed these reductions in mortality in conjunction with publish-

Annual deaths per 100,000
U.S. population aged ≥ 15

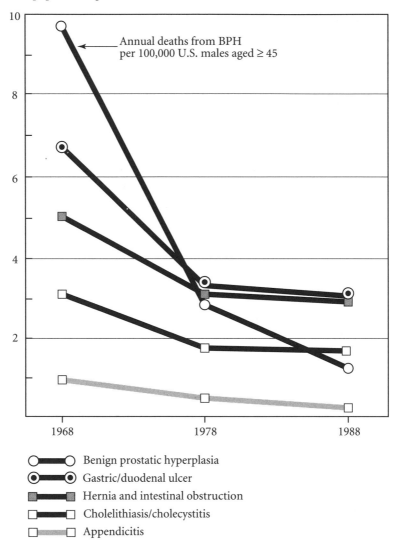

Annual deaths from BPH
per 100,000 U.S. males aged ≥ 45

⊖━━⊖ Benign prostatic hyperplasia
◉━━◉ Gastric/duodenal ulcer
■━━■ Hernia and intestinal obstruction
☐━━☐ Cholelithiasis/cholecystitis
☐━━☐ Appendicitis

ed NCHS estimates based on samples from the National Hospital Discharge Survey on rates of inpatient hospitalization for the diseases studied and rates of surgical procedures performed for the same population during the years studied.

Appendicitis. For the treatment of appendicitis, both hospitalization and surgery rates have declined over the twenty-year period (see Figure 16-3): we found an 18 percent decrease in the annual rate of hospitalization for appendicitis among persons aged 15 and over in U.S. hospitals between 1968 and 1978, and a further 20 percent decrease between 1978 and 1988, as well as a parallel 11 percent decline in the appendectomy rate between 1968 and 1978, and 14 percent from 1978 to 1988 [3]. We attribute these declining rates to improvements in diagnostic techniques, training of surgeons, and antibiotic therapy, factors that have also contributed to the decreasing rates of mortality and length of hospital stay shown in Figures 16-1 and 16-2.

Gallbladder disease. It has been estimated that approximately 12 percent of the adult population in the United States is probably carrying gallstones, and that the national cost for gallbladder operations exceeds $3 billion annually [2]. While the rate of hospitalization for gallbladder disease remained relatively constant between 1968 and 1978, it decreased 17 percent from 1978 to 1988. The rate of cholecystectomy (gallbladder removal), in contrast, remained almost constant during this decade, after having been nearly halved during the period 1968–1978 (see Figure 16-4).

Figure 16-1. Changes in mortality rates for surgically treated diseases. The decline in mortality over a twenty-year period, as reported by the National Center for Health Statistics (NCHS), for five surgically treated conditions among patients in U.S. hospitals. Annual rates are per 100,000 males aged 45 and over for benign prostatic hyperplasia, and per 100,000 males and females aged 15 and over for the other diseases. Deaths from benign prostatic hyperplasia declined 69 percent from 1968 to 1978 and 54 percent between 1978 and 1988. There was a 50 percent reduction in mortality from gastric and duodenal ulcer from 1968 to 1978, but little change in the subsequent decade. The death rate from hernia and intestinal obstruction decreased 40 percent from 1968 to 1978, but only slightly from 1978 to 1988, and mortality from gallbladder disease (cholelithiasis/cholecystitis) followed the same pattern. The annual rate of mortality from appendicitis decreased 60 percent between 1968 and 1978 and 43 percent between 1978 and 1988. (Reproduced with permission from Milamed and Hedley-White [3].)

Average LOS (days), all ages

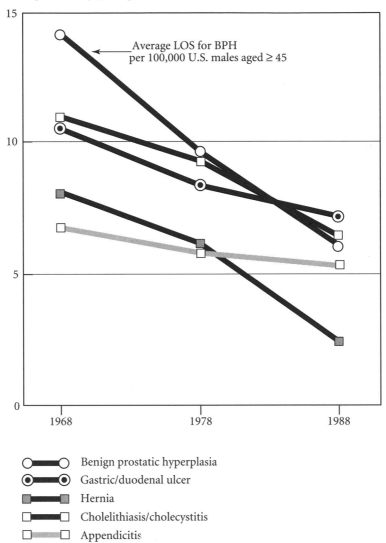

In 1934, Heuer estimated that the mortality for surgery of the gallbladder was 6.6 percent. The apparent rate of mortality from all causes during hospitalization for all cholecystectomy cases was 0.07 percent in 1978, falling to 0.06 percent in 1988, an apparent 99 percent decrease in fifty years [2, 3]. The NCHS has noted that cholecystectomies among patients aged 65 and older rose from 399 per 100,000 population annually in 1965 to 570 in 1986, while the rate for all ages did not change significantly. At present, an increasing number of cholecystectomies are done using laparoscopic techniques, thus further reducing the length of hospitalization (see Chapter 3).

Gastric and duodenal ulcer. Operations such as vagotomy and drainage, vagotomy and antrectomy, vagotomy and hemigastrectomy—in general terms, severing a portion of the vagus nerve and removing parts of the stomach—were once widely used in the treatment of gastric and duodenal ulcer. As Figure 16-5 shows, advances in medical therapy, such as the use of histamine-2 blockers (see Chapter 14), have reduced both the need for surgery and inpatient hospitalization [3].

In 1983, Doctors Warren and Marshall of the Royal Perth Hospital in Western Australia reported the presence of a small, S-shaped bacillus in specimens from patients undergoing gastroscopy and biopsy for gastritis. It has since been determined that this Gram-negative, microaerophilic bacillus, which was given the name *Helicobacter pylori,* is present in nearly

---

Figure 16-2. Average length of hospital stay (LOS) for patients with surgically treated diseases. The length of hospital stay (LOS), or days of inpatient hospitalization, from 1968 to 1978 and 1978 to 1988 decreased for patients with primary diagnoses of five diseases treated by surgery. NCHS data are for patients of all ages in U.S. hospitals, but for males aged 45 and over in the case of benign prostatic hyperplasia. The average length of stay for appendicitis remained relatively constant while technological advances resulted in 33 percent reductions over each decade for patients with benign prostate hyperplasia. We attribute the 58 percent reduction in length of hospital stay from 1978 to 1988 for patients with hernia to advances that presently allow much surgical hernia repair to be performed on an outpatient basis. Nonsurgical treatment of gastric and duodenal ulcer has greatly reduced days of inpatient hospitalization for this condition, while advances in patient monitoring and the use of laparoscopic techniques have shortened the average stay for gallbladder disease.

Annual discharges from U.S. hospitals
per 100,000 population aged ≥ 15

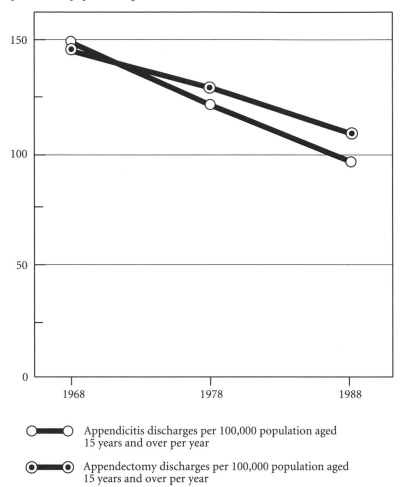

○━━━○ Appendicitis discharges per 100,000 population aged
15 years and over per year

◉━━━◉ Appendectomy discharges per 100,000 population aged
15 years and over per year

Figure 16-3. Rate of hospitalization for appendicitis and appendectomy. The rate of inpatient hospitalization for appendicitis among patients aged 15 and over in U.S. hospitals decreased 18 percent from 1968 to 1978, 20 percent between 1978 and 1988. The annual rate of appendectomy decreased 11 percent between 1968 and 1978 and 14 percent from 1978 to 1988. For the years 1978 and 1988, the rates of appendectomy exceed slightly the rates for hospitalization with appendicitis as primary diagnosis. (Reproduced with permission from Milamed and Hedley-White [3].)

Annual discharges from U.S. hospitals
per 100,000 population aged ≥ 15

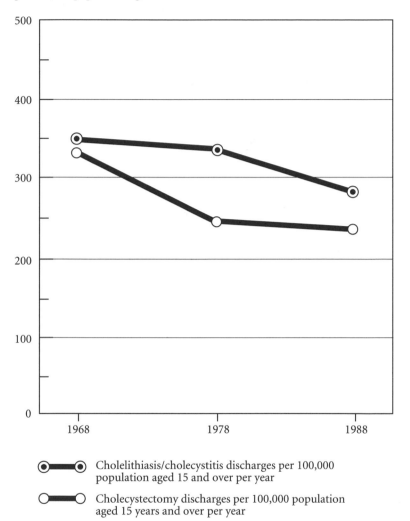

Figure 16-4. Rate of hospitalization for cholelithiasis/cholecystitis and cholecystectomy. Patients in United States hospitals aged 15 years and over with gallbladder disease were hospitalized at a rate that remained nearly constant between 1968 and 1978 but that dropped 17 percent between 1978 and 1988. The rate of cholecystectomy for the same population decreased 23 percent between 1968 and 1978 but remained stable from 1978 to 1988. Because the numbers of cholecystectomies reported were combined with other biliary tract procedures in 1968, the actual decrease from 1968 to 1978 may be less than that shown. (Reproduced with permission from Milamed and Hedley-White [3].)

Annual discharges from U.S. hospitals
per 100,000 population aged ≥ 15

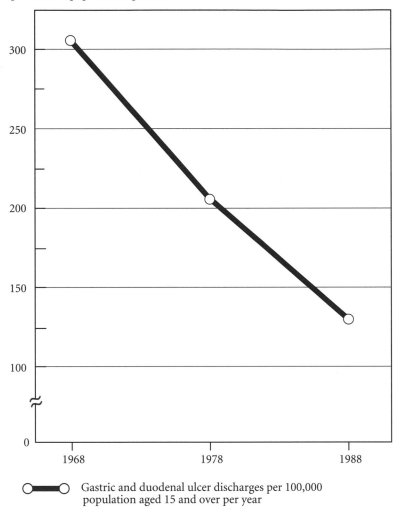

<O━━━O> Gastric and duodenal ulcer discharges per 100,000
population aged 15 and over per year

Figure 16-5. Rate of hospitalization for gastric and duodenal ulcer. The decline is sharp in the annual rate of hospitalization for gastric and duodenal ulcer among patients aged 15 and over in U.S. hospitals: 32 percent between 1968 and 1978 and 39 percent from 1978 to 1988. (Reproduced with permission from Milamed and Hedley-White [3].)

all patients with duodenal ulcer and approximately 80 percent of those with gastric ulcer. However, *H. pylori* is also found, to a lesser extent, in the epithelium lining the digestive tract in healthy persons, and its prevalence increases with age. Over the past decade researchers have reached a consensus that this microbe is a major causative factor in the development of gastritis and gastric and duodenal ulcer. In February of 1994 a panel of experts assembled by the National Institutes of Health (NIH) determined that there was a definite connection between infection with *H. pylori* and ulcers. By treating this infection instead of only the symptoms, the panel concluded, the rate of recurrence of peptic ulcer disease could be reduced by 90 percent or more. It also came to a consensus decision on ulcer therapy: a recommendation for testing for *H. pylori* of all patients with ulcer disease or a history of this condition. All those with test results showing *H. pylori* infection should receive two weeks of antibiotic treatment. Hospital discharges for this condition decreased by a third between 1968 and 1978 and further decreased 39 percent between 1978 and 1988. The reduction in hospital use resulted from this shift to nonsurgical therapies. Mortality due to gastric and duodenal ulcer was reduced by one-half between 1968 and 1978, but remained almost constant between 1978 and 1988 [3] (see Figure 16-1). Over the twenty-year period studied, length of hospital stay was reduced from an average of 10.7 days to 7.2 (see Figure 16-2).

Hernia and intestinal obstruction. Rates of hospitalization for hernia and intestinal obstruction are illustrated together because data on mortality from these causes combined are available for comparison. The most common form of intestinal obstruction results when a portion of the small intestine becomes pinched off by untreated hernia. The annual rate of inpatient hospitalization for hernia remained nearly constant between 1968 and 1978 but was halved between 1978 and 1988 (see Figure 16-6). Over this twenty-year period, the annual rate for surgical hernia repair as an inpatient hospital procedure fell 44 percent. We attribute this decrease to the introduction during the period 1978–1988 of outpatient hernia repair not reflected in NCHS discharge data for inpatient procedures [3]. This change also underlies the drastic reduction in average length of hospital stay reported for hernia (see Figure 16-2). Mortality from hernia and intestinal obstruction decreased 40 percent between 1968 and 1988 [3] (see Figure 16-1).

Annual discharges from U.S. hospitals
per 100,000 population aged ≥ 15

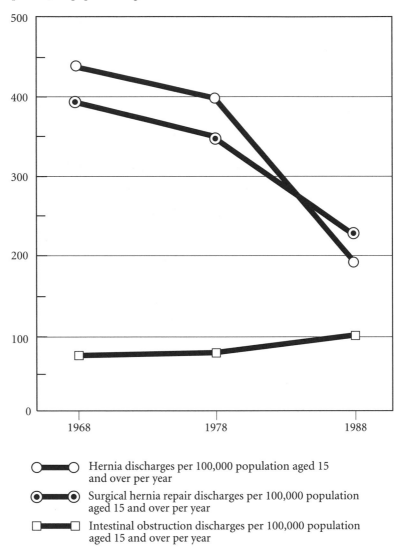

○━━○ Hernia discharges per 100,000 population aged 15
and over per year

◉━━◉ Surgical hernia repair discharges per 100,000 population
aged 15 and over per year

▫━━▫ Intestinal obstruction discharges per 100,000 population
aged 15 and over per year

Because many surgical procedures used in the treatment of intestinal obstruction have other applications, such as resection to treat malignancies, we were unable to derive rates of surgery for this diagnosis. The published estimates of numbers of surgical procedures from NCHS do not identify the primary diagnoses for which they were performed. Figure 16-6 shows a modest increase from 1968 to 1988 in hospitalization for intestinal obstruction [3].

Benign prostate hyperplasia. In 1983 prostatectomy was the most frequently performed urological procedure and the tenth most common operation in the United States [7]. The rate of hospitalization for benign prostate hyperplasia (BPH) among U.S. males aged 45 and over increased 24 percent between 1968 and 1978 and decreased 15 percent between 1978 and 1988 (see Figure 16-7), while the rate of surgery of the prostate increased 23.2 percent from 1968 to 1988. At the same time mortality decreased tenfold [3] (see Figure 16-1), and average length of hospital stay was reduced by more than half (see Figure 16-2). We attribute this major reduction in mortality to a number of factors, which include improved training of urologists, advances in anesthesiology, better management of blood and electrolyte loss, improved postoperative nursing and care, advances in cardiology such as presurgery evaluation and treatment of coronary artery disease, and the mandatory use of pulse oximetry, a noninvasive but accurate means of measuring blood oxygenation during surgery. This reduction in mortality is especially significant. Men over the age of 65 in the United States have a rate of prostatectomy 2.3 times higher than that for all U.S. males aged 45 and over, and the number of males in this age group continues to increase.

Figure 16-6. Rate of hospitalization for hernia, hernia repair, and intestinal obstruction. Little changes in the rate of hospitalization for hernia among patients aged 15 and over in U.S. hospitals between 1968 and 1978, but there was a dramatic decline of 52 percent from 1978 to 1988. The rate for surgical hernia repair (herniorrhaphy) among the same population decreased in parallel between 1968 and 1978, but it dropped 37 percent from 1978 to 1988 because of the trend to outpatient herniorrhaphy. We were unable to derive rates for surgical treatment of intestinal obstruction, but hospitalizations with intestinal obstruction as a primary diagnosis increased 10 percent from 1968 to 1978 and 18 percent from 1978 to 1988. (Reproduced with permission from Milamed and Hedley-White [3].)

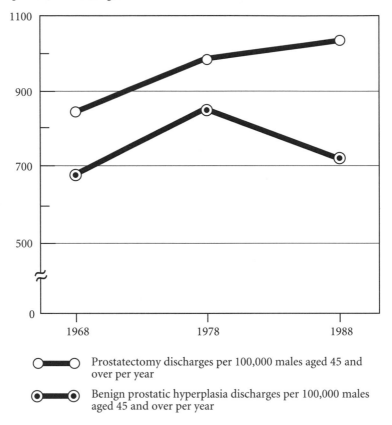

Annual discharges from U.S. hospitals
per 100,000 males aged ≥ 45

⊶⊶○ Prostatectomy discharges per 100,000 males aged 45 and
over per year

⊙⊶⊙ Benign prostatic hyperplasia discharges per 100,000 males
aged 45 and over per year

Figure 16-7. Rate of hospitalization for benign prostatic hyperplasia and pro-statectomy. The annual rate of hospitalization for benign prostatic hyperplasia among males aged 45 and over in U.S. hospitals increased by a quarter from 1968 to 1978 and decreased 15 percent from 1978 to 1988. Among the same population the rate of prostatectomy or prostate surgery increased 27 percent from 1968 to 1978 and then remained relatively constant. These modest increases in surgery and inpatient treatment must be interpreted in the light of the dramatic declines in mortality and length of patient stay illustrated in Figures 16-1 and 16-2. (Reproduced with permission from Milamed and Hedley-White [3].)

Manpower and Technology in Health Care

We have reviewed the reduction in mortality attributable to five common diseases treatable by surgery over the twenty-year period 1968 to 1988 because we consider it the most meaningful measure of the contributions of surgery, anesthesiology, and related disciplines. Changing trends in health care manpower, the growth of specialized professional societies and promulgation of standards in health care, technological advances, improved monitoring and care of patients during surgery and the perioperative period, and the increasing presence of intensive care units have played important roles in the reduction of mortality. In addition, a complex array of nontechnological variables have probably contributed to the decline in deaths, but socioeconomic factors such as the accessibility of medical care, increased insurance coverage, better education, nutrition, housing and environmental quality are beyond the scope of this chapter.

Health care manpower. According to the American Medical Association, the number of anesthesiologists per 100,000 U.S. population more than doubled during the period 1965–1989, while the number of surgeons increased only 10 percent, and radiologists declined [3]. Between 1971 and 1988 the membership of the American Society of Anesthesiologists increased more than 100 percent [3]. According to the American Hospital Association, the number of full-time employed registered nurses increased 43 percent between 1978 and 1988 [3]. While membership in professional societies is not an accurate measure of active employment, nursing societies specializing in perioperative and intensive care saw tremendous growth from 1967 to 1989. Membership in the American Association of Critical Care Nurses increased from its 140 founding members in 1969 to almost 70,000 by 1988, and the American Association of Post-Anesthesia Care Nurses grew from its initial 900 members in 1980 to 4,500 in 1988 [3].

Standards of practice. In health care as in all fields, a major contribution of specialized professional societies and academic training programs and research has been the development and promulgation of standards of practice. In medicine, general standards outlining processes and recommendations rather than actual clinical protocols have predominated. An example of the development of standards is provided by Eichhorn and colleagues from the Anesthesia Department at Harvard Medical School [8]. Harvard Medical School's Anesthesia Department, based in nine teaching hospitals, has been insured by Harvard's own malpractice insurance company. When this insurer approached the heads of the hospitals' Anesthesia Departments about the number of anesthesia-related accidents and claims from 1976 to 1984, they established a risk management committee of senior anesthesiologists to study the matter. After analyzing information from the insurance company's incident files, the committee believed that most of the anesthesia-related incidents recorded by the insurer that had resulted in death or major morbidity could have been prevented, and concluded that improved patient monitoring would decrease the number of accidents. The committee felt that the issuing of *mandatory* standards for patient monitoring, rather than the more typical "guidelines" or "recommended practices," was in keeping with the magnitude of the concerns addressed. The standards were developed with the goals of improving patient care and the detection of infrequent adverse events, providing an objective means of evaluation, and "to establish a precedent" [8].

The original standards for minimal monitoring adopted in 1985 included the mandatory presence of an anesthesiologist or nurse anesthetist in the operating room throughout the course of the anesthetic, arterial blood pressure and heart rate measurement at five-minute intervals, continuous electrocardiogram display, continuous monitoring of ventilation and circulation, continuous monitoring of potential disconnection of the breathing system, continuous analysis of the oxygen within the patient breathing system, and a readily available means of patient temperature measurement [8].

Adoption of these standards resulted in an approximately threefold decrease in serious anesthesia-related accidents involving low-risk patients in the Harvard Medical School hospital system during the period 1985–1988. Shortly after the adoption of these mandatory standards, Harvard Medical School's insurer began to reduce premium increases for insured anesthesiologists, until in 1988 premiums actually decreased 5 percent [9]. The American Society of Anesthesiolgists has adopted standards for the monitoring of patients during surgery and the postoperative period based on the Harvard standards outlined above [10].

The Association of Operating Room Nurses (AORN) published its first *Standards of Nursing Practice* in 1975. In subsequent years the scope of these standards has expanded to include such topics as patient monitoring, radiological safety, sterilization, professional performance, and patient outcomes. The Association for the Advancement of Medical Instrumentation (AAMI) and the American Society for Testing and Materials (ASTM) publish annual compendia of standards and recommended practices.

Advances in patient monitoring and intensive care instrumentation. During the decade 1968–1978 the use of arterial blood gas monitoring became widespread, facilitating the management of perioperative respiratory failure. During the 1980s, the use of pulse oximetry, or the continuous measurement of blood oxygenation by measuring the absorbance of light passing through a body tissue, typically a finger, provided the anesthesiologist with continuous data. The perioperative measurement of arterial carbon dioxide was greatly enhanced by the use of the capnometer. These technical advances in monitoring have enhanced the effectiveness of the standards of practice described earlier. The capital costs of the equipment used in the average operating room have increased fivefold in recent years. At the same time, the American Society for Testing and Materials' Committee F-29 on Anesthetic and Respiratory Equipment and the International Organization for Standardization's Technical Committee 121 on Anaesthesia and Respiratory Equipment have greatly expanded their activity in the development and publication of internationally accepted, voluntary consensus performance standards, intended to assure the utility and reliability of this equipment.

Development of the intensive care unit. The assignment of critically ill or other patients who need extra attention from nursing staff to general hospital wards results in increased personnel requirements for these wards. The shortage of nursing personnel in the United States after World War II prompted hospitals to establish surgical recovery rooms to provide more cost effective, specialized nursing care [11]. By 1960, surgical recovery rooms were found in almost all United States hospitals. The intensive care unit was modeled on the success and wide acceptance of the recovery room. The Office of Technology Assessment's study of intensive care units [11] attributes the increase in these special care facilities after the late 1950s to the more widespread use of mechanical ventilators. These life-support devices were most efficiently monitored from a central location. Approximately 80 percent of short-term general hospitals in the United States had intensive care units by the early 1980s. At present there is increasing specialization of the intensive care unit in the areas of cardiac care, trauma, and surgical and medical intensive care.

Advances in information transfer. During the decade 1978–1988 advances in information transfer in operating rooms and intensive care units and the increased use of computerized patient records have contributed to the improvement of perioperative care. Computerized patient record systems provide physicians, nurses, and other personnel with immediate access to laboratory data of all kinds—hematology, blood gas, pathology—as well as vital patient history information, such as medications taken and allergies.

Ambulatory surgery. Advances in perioperative care coupled with incentives for cost containment have resulted in reductions in length of hospital stay (see Figure 16-2). The same complex of factors underlies the growing trend toward ambulatory surgery. The terms "ambulatory surgery" and "outpatient surgery" are often used interchangeably to refer to surgical procedures performed without inpatient hospital admission. "Outpatient surgery," however, most often denotes procedures that are performed without hospital admission and that involve local anesthesia, if any, with immediate discharge of the patient. "Ambulatory surgery" is usually defined as surgery requiring a postoperative recovery period after local, regional, or general anesthesia, with the patient discharged the same day.

In the 1970s ambulatory surgery became widely accepted because of the potential for cost savings and patient convenience. By 1982 approximately 70 percent of nonfederal hospitals located in major metropolitan areas of the United States offered ambulatory surgery, and there were approximately 250 separate, "free-standing" ambulatory surgery facilities not affiliated with hospitals as well [12]. According to American Hospital Association data, in 1980 outpatient or ambulatory surgery accounted for 16 percent of all hospital surgeries performed, and by 1990 this proportion had increased to 51 percent. By 1988 there were more than 1,000 free-standing ambulatory surgical facilities in the United States.

During the early 1980s, it had been estimated that between 20 and 40 percent of all surgical procedures could be performed on an ambulatory basis. Later estimates, taking into account advances in laser technology, fiber optics (endoscopy), and anesthesia, run as high as 60 percent [12]. Although a wide range of procedures are performed in hospital ambulatory surgery units and independent surgery centers, the American Medical Association has emphasized the importance of assessing the needs of the individual patient when determining the most appropriate surgical setting.

At this time, repair of inguinal hernia became one of the most common surgical procedures performed on an ambulatory basis. Many herniorrhaphy procedures require only local anesthesia, and by the time of hospital discharge the patient is expected to be alert and fully ambulatory. Alternatively, postoperative problems such as urinary retention and wound complications may develop, necessitating adequate patient education and physician follow-up. While elimination of pre- and postoperative hospital stay reduces hospital charges, it is difficult to quantify the costs of home care provided.

Conclusion

The reduction in mortality over time for several conditions most often treated by surgery is the most meaningful measure of progress in surgery, anesthesiology, and perioperative care. Global factors affecting trends in morbidity and mortality are many and complex. We have directed the readers' attention to some of the most significant developments affecting perioperative care during the past twenty-five years, though we cannot quantify the contributions of individual technologies to the positive results we have demonstrated. Advances in surgery, anesthesiology, and related technologies continue to reduce mortality and length of hospital stay for patients treated by surgery.

At the same time, increasing costs necessitate ongoing detailed study of the role of surgery in contemporary American medicine. As new surgical techniques and methodologies are developed, the need for quantitative instruments to assess their risks and benefits increases. The trend toward "major" ambulatory surgery mandates further prospective studies of patient outcome. Advances in the collection and classification of hospital utilization data, and the forthcoming expansion of NCHS hospital discharge data to include outpatient diagnoses and procedures, will help assure continued progress.

Editors' Note

Increased understanding of the mechanisms and processes of disease, and increased capacity to intervene, paradoxically have increased the complexity of the clinical response to disease. The development of modern surgery is a case in point. Mastery of the relevant knowledge and the appropriate responses needed to treat a patient is no longer the province of a single individual; rather, treatment requires a team, each member of which has a specialized function. Reciprocally, this specialization of work aids and supports the elaboration of even more specialized technologies. Examples include transfusion therapy, critical care nursing, mandatory standards for anesthesia, and the use of heart-lung machines.

The improvements in surgical outcomes noted in this chapter result from advances made in a variety of fields—from the invention of new instruments for less invasive surgery to more stringent standards of monitoring the administration of anesthesia, from basic research into bacterial infection to the increasing use of intensive care units for postoperative patients. Just as it is necessary to evaluate the efficacy and cost-effectiveness of a new device or drug, we must also measure the benefits and costs of new settings for delivering care, such as independent ambulatory surgery centers. The assessment of such administrative innovations, illustrated by this chapter, will become even more important as the health care system becomes more complex.

PART J

Conclusions and Recommendations

17

Improving the Health Care System

FREDERICK MOSTELLER AND HOWARD S. FRAZIER

Background

The case studies of medical innovations presented in this book bring together a wealth of information about different technologies and practices in modern medicine. Taken together, these various detailed analyses have led us to a number of policy lessons and recommendations with respect to our system of health care as a whole. One common thread in these cases, for example, is the importance of measuring the effects of each innovation so that our decisions to adopt or not adopt it are based on solid information about benefits and financial and social costs.

No small series of cases can illustrate more than a fraction of the issues we must address, however. In this chapter we discuss recommendations of broad scope that emerge only indirectly from the cases. Each has been selected on the basis of three characteristics: it is the object of current development efforts; implementation of a recommended policy is not dependent upon any specific configuration of reforms of our system of health care; and each recommendation strengthens technology assessment almost independent of the nature of the technology. Finally, because we highly value randomized, controlled trials and evidence-based medicine, we focus on ideas that have prospects of increasing the number of clinical trials and strengthening the evidential foundation of medical practice.

In brief, we explore in this chapter several goals for the health care system as a whole: (1) improving organization and dissemination of the results of clinical trials; (2) increasing the number and size of trials; (3) improving post-marketing surveillance; (4) encouraging hospitals to evaluate, on a regular basis, the care they deliver; (5) improving economic analyses of treatment and of technology assessment; (6) summarizing the contributions of medicine to quality of life; and (7) giving thoughtful consideration to the role of clinical trials and medical technology assessment in our own, individual health care. We will consider here in more detail some steps that might be taken that would not attempt to revolutionize the health care system but would make more effective the medical care that is delivered. These proposed steps would not necessarily reduce the total bill—that requires massive overhaul—but they would deliver more medical support for a dollar spent.

Different readers will find different points of agreement with our recommendations. As patients they may be pleased to know of beneficial developments and be able to take advantage of some of them. As advocates they may wish to encourage some of these innovations. Those participating in making health or insurance policy will want to improve the system of gathering and disseminating information of value to caregivers.

This book is about what works in medicine and how we know what works. Therefore we stress the appropriate use of the kinds of information discussed here. As our first suggestion for improving health care, we advise taking more advantage of the information that has already been gathered.

Organizing Medical Knowledge

As we mentioned in Chapter 2, the field of obstetrics is unique in that the results of all the known clinical trials have been gathered, organized, and analyzed by a group centered at Oxford University. This effort took quite a few years to accomplish: all the organizations that were carrying out randomized or quasi-randomized clinical trials had to be located, their investigations registered, and the progress and outcomes of the research recorded.

Once this had been done, teams were formed to analyze the data. Often many studies of the same or almost the same medical question were carried out, and differences in outcome were discovered. In the face of disagreement serious efforts must be made to carry out a synthesis of the research. Over the last fifteen years considerable progress has been made in creating objective methods for carrying out such syntheses, though they require considerable time and money as well as technical expertise. The teams that prepared the summaries for obstetrics carried out overviews (meta-analyses) in standard ways, and the data base has been gathered and put on electronic systems and made available so that others can update the analyses or carry out new analyses as may seem useful.

It had been the dream of a distinguished British medical researcher, Archie Cochrane, that all the clinical trials carried out in medicine would be gathered together and suitably analyzed and updated. Although this work has been carried out for obstetrics [1, 2], so far it has not been done for the rest of medicine. Nevertheless, there is now a substantial movement, led by Iain Chalmers at the UK Cochrane Centre, to organize the results of all kinds of studies. Its goal is to gather all the randomized trials currently in the literature and keep track of the progress made through new studies. Enthusiasm for this program has been substantial and a number of research centers throughout the world have asked that they be named UK Cochrane Centre affiliates to help with this gigantic task. When completed, the findings will be an invaluable addition to the medical armamentarium.

Why can't physicians do this work themselves? The effort is overwhelming. Somewhere between five and ten thousand randomized trials are carried out each year. Experts reviewing the literature have to find the research papers on each topic and analyze them. These tasks alone take much time and effort, including specialized training. Although physicians will learn a lot by participating in the venture (and many will), their primary job of caring for patients leaves relatively little time available for research. Lack of time, lack of resources, and lack of training are serious obstacles for practicing physicians. They need material that has been summarized for them in ready, usable form.

Once this material is organized, we will be much further along the path toward knowing what medical treatments work better than others. Of course, new treatments will always be introduced, and they in turn will need evaluation and comparison with other technologies, and so we are talking about a continuous process. Thus, not only must we bring our knowledge up to the state of the art, we also need to establish a system that keeps us informed of cutting-edge research. Because people like to participate in new things, a system of continual updating may be harder to establish than the initial effort to gather the baseline information. In any case, the first step would be to organize the baseline information—a summary of what research has already been done—and this information must be digested and kept available for alternative analyses.

When this effort has been carried out, we will have a much better idea of what we know and don't know about medicine, not only the merits of treatments but also the general practice of medicine. Once we gain an overview of available knowledge as a whole, we should see more clearly what additional evaluative efforts have the best chance of improving the health of the nation.

To illustrate the kinds of findings that an organization of information can produce, consider the summaries offered by the obstetric studies cited in the book *Guide to Effective Care in Pregnancy and Child Birth* [3]. This book lists about 175 forms of care that reduce negative outcomes in pregnancy and child birth, such as reducing smoking during pregnancy, reducing the likelihood of low-birth-weight babies, and preventing measles after birth by vaccination. It also notes scores of promising procedures that have not yet proved themselves and need to be evaluated further, such as the use of folate supplements or the administration of prostaglandins to induce labor. The *Guide* also identifies treatments that some investigators have recommended but that as yet are supported by little available evidence, as well as about a hundred procedures that are regarded as having negative value and that should be abandoned.

Additional Sources of Clinical Trials

We should gather the data that are already available and make the most of them—the investigations have been carried out, and only analyzing and editing the materials is required to make them more useful. Of course, other questions then arise: what additional studies are needed, and how should new studies be carried out? Programs for guiding the direction of new research have been proposed and are in progress. Perhaps the simplest of the proposals to describe is that by Richard Peto of the United Kingdom. His idea is that we need more clinical trials—randomized trials—but that they need to be larger and simpler.

Why do they need to be simpler? The two main reasons are cost and generality of inference. When we take down all the details of every patient's life, including many pieces of information that a hospital might not ordinarily collect, we make the research project both more complicated and more costly. The interviewing itself, then the storage and analysis of the information, takes up the time of the investigators and also time with the patient, who may not be in very good shape for giving information. If we collect as little information as we can get along with, the study itself will be considerably less expensive to carry out.

Does this not mean that there is a danger that we will not collect some fact that will turn out to be important? Yes, but this risk arises in every investigation. There is always the possibility that science will discover some new variable whose absence from a previous study may ultimately make the findings less valuable than they at first seemed.

Fortunately and unfortunately, such variables do not come along very often. It is fortunate because we do not care to have our studies destroyed by the introduction of variables previously unknown or considered irrelevant. New variables are rare because medicine has been studied for a long time; except at the frontiers of research, we do not expect them to interfere with clinical studies. Once in a while they do, as when a totally new form of treatment, such as antibiotics, is introduced. Unfortunately, we do not often get an entirely new treatment that has great effect, but when we do it is a matter for celebration. We are expecting much to develop in the next few years from the new work in genetics and the studies of molecular biology.

By not collecting so much data, we can lower the costs of studies. In addition, though, we can also hope to enroll more patients in the investigations. Fewer patients would be ineligible to participate in the trials. We would have large trials but they would sample as nearly as possible from the total population of patients subject to the disease under study. To the extent that this is possible, patients and society benefit in two ways.

First, the patients would represent the whole population of those needing treatment. Often trials are used to study special sets of people who do not have any additional disabilities besides those being studied in the trial. For example, older people are likely to suffer from several troubles and so they are often barred from participation in trials on the grounds that the investigators want to know whether the treatment is successful under ideal conditions. Does it work? After that is determined, then we might ask whether it works under average conditions or for most conditions. By including all kinds of patients in the trial, we would learn whether the treatment works well for all patients under a variety of conditions.

Furthermore, when the trial is large we have the further opportunity to examine the issue of effectiveness of the treatment in differing subgroups. For example, some diseases progress in stages, and the question arises whether a treatment has any benefit at the various stages of the disease. Similarly, is the treatment beneficial when given to patients who suffer not only from the basic disease but also from additional afflictions?

Thus the large, simple trial saves money by gathering comparatively less information and offers the possibility of being generalized to the whole population of patients. It also enables investigators to compare the effectiveness of the treatment in subgroups of patients.

One way to make medical experimentation more feasible is to make it cheaper and to make it more readily generalizable to the public to be treated. Through increased size we make it possible to study the differences in performance of a treatment in subgroups of the population, such as people of various ages, those with various degrees of severity of disease, or those with other medical problems.

Post-Marketing Surveillance

Although randomized comparative trials of therapies provide good evidence of their value, ordinarily we cannot expect that trials will last long enough to detect effects that are slow in developing or be large enough to detect rare side effects. For example, side effects that appear a decade or so after treatment will not likely be detected in a clinical trial.

To help detect rare or slow-developing effects, we need a back-up for the clinical trial, one that might be based upon a registry or on a post-marketing system. Currently we have a post-marketing system that is weak. Essentially, the physician who notices an adverse side effect (of a drug or certain devices) is supposed to tell the FDA or the manufacturer, and the manufacturer is supposed to report to the FDA.

One advantage post-marketing monitoring offers is that many more patients will be treated by the medication than would have been involved in a clinical trial. Another advantage is that the surveillance can encompass years or even decades. The disadvantages are parallel to the advantages: the physician may not recognize the need to report a side effect, for example. Making a connection between an outcome and a treatment given long ago is not easy, and at best uncertain. Even when the physician is aware of the treatment, the effect may not be reported because the chance of the relation being causal rather than accidental may seem remote to the physician. The physician does not want to stir up turmoil for no reason. Thus the likelihood of strong reporting based on voluntary recognition is not high.

In the United Kingdom, a somewhat different approach has been used with good effect. Over a period of time, concerns are gathered that certain drugs may be causing adverse side effects. From a central office a letter goes out to physicians asking for outcome information for specific patients who have been given certain prescriptions. The physician is asked to review the patients who have taken a medication and report on outcome. In this way a basis for looking into rumors is established (see Chapter 15 for additional information).

Probably we could have a similar activity in this country, at least for prescriptions that were given to patients in the Medicare system. The whole country need not be involved in every inquiry. Sample survey methods could be used to make the reviews economical. We must keep in mind the costliness of a procedure that asks a physician to spend time reviewing records, often of substantial numbers of patients. Under the British system the physician is being paid for his or her time, whether it is spent on reporting records or taking care of patients. Under our system, the self-employed physician would be adding an unpaid task to his or her work unless a fee were paid for such reports; in a health maintenance organization with salaried physicians, the time would have to be paid for by either the requesting agency or the employing organization. It would be wise to carry out a cost-effectiveness analysis for any surveillance system before trying to launch it.

"The Firm": Organizing Hospitals for Trials

Another idea for developing comparative investigations of treatments and diagnoses in medicine sails under the name of "the firm." The basic idea is that every institution should be investigating its own performance in delivering good health care. It should be able to evaluate costs, risks, and benefits of the therapies it delivers for common conditions. Indeed, in principle, each physician should be trying to do the same for the patients in his or her practice. A physician with a highly varied practice might find evaluation difficult, because so few cases of one kind are available for comparison. For the same reason, hospitals may not be able to assess themselves very well for their handling of rare conditions.

In the way we ordinarily run clinical trials, it takes a large effort in time and money as well as expertise to set one up. The question arises whether such heavy developmental effort is required or whether this is not something that should be routine in every fair-sized institution. It may not be very practical in the case of a particular physician's practice, depending upon the kind of practice. Physicians have traditionally followed series of cases that have been treated in a similar manner and have reported the results of the treatments when they felt they had enough data. Chapter 3 illustrates a report of a series for gallbladder operations (see Tables 3-1 and 3-2).

Though we prefer as patients to think that we are being given sure-fire, well-investigated treatments, what we read in the newspapers and see and hear through the media shows us that changes in medicine occur every day and that new findings mean that old ways will become obsolete—perhaps not right away, but after a while. We are all involved in a great continuing investigation of how to get the most that medicine can offer. We prefer not to use the word *experiment* here, because experimentation means not just observing outcomes but also control by the investigator of conditions and treatment delivered. Thus experimentation implies more control than physicians ordinarily have when they treat patients as they appear in practice.

Physician reports of this kind are called "observational studies," and it is more difficult to reach firm conclusions about causation from these studies than from controlled experiments. And that is why we want the results of the many controlled experiments in medicine gathered, organized, and analyzed. Of course, the kinds of observations physicians make in practical circumstances when joined with information from the biological sciences lead to new treatments and to controlled investigations.

The concept of "the firm" is used to suggest the organizational structure and evaluation practices, or bookkeeping, of business firms. Institutions such as hospitals might be arranged so that they can almost automatically investigate questions intended to lead to improvements in health care within their own institution. We would also encourage hospitals to be organized so that they are able to contribute to medicine generally by being ready to participate in studies of multi-institutional issues [4–6]. Readiness to carry out such studies is partly a matter of attitude, not just a matter of competence or funding. For example, the physicians at a hospital may want to know whether certain ways of carrying out treatments are better than others. These need not be earthshaking issues, but merely choices among two or more ways of doing things that are equally easy or equally expensive but that may have different pay-offs.

The thought behind recommending that hospitals be organized in this way is that if an institution is ready to do comparative experiments on short notice, it will be ready to join in the effort to evaluate medicine in the year 2000. A similar situation existed early in the century in the field of public opinion polls. It used to be very difficult to carry out a national public opinion poll, but because business and industry and the news media wanted such information, economic pressure caused the development of a number of commercial public opinion polls. Soon it became possible to complete a national poll—which formerly took months or years to develop, carry out, and analyze—in a few days, or in extremity even hours. Interviews and clinical trials are studies that differ considerably in the time required, but the time required *to get ready* to do either depends on the presence or absence of an organization in readiness.

This idea of a medical institution ready to carry out experimental investigations is drawn from the idea of the firm. Studies require at least two comparable groups. It is possible for a hospital of adequate size to divide itself into two, three, four, or more comparable groups called firms. Each group has essentially the same number of beds, the same access to ICU units, the same size nursing staff, the same composition of physicians, and the same source of pharmaceuticals. The patients entering the institution are assigned to one of the firms at random, and they then belong to that firm.

As nearly as possible the several firms are equivalent. Consequently, if a question arises as to the preferability of a particular way of handling patients of a specific type, it is possible to treat those in Firm A in one manner, those in Firm B in another, and so on. At the close of the investigation, we would have samples of comparable patients (because of the randomization) treated in different ways by comparable firms. We would then be able to carry out controlled experiments.

Many of the kinds of questions that need to be studied in this way are local in their importance, and yet they make a difference to the institution and its staff. When people ask whether one plan or another is better for carrying out a particular mission, it is well to have a means of responding to the question. If it turns out that a choice between two options makes no difference to patient outcome, all the better—just knowing that is helpful.

In sum, the idea of the firm has two important aspects. First, the local one—an institution organized into firms can carry out comparative studies about matters of special interest to it. The second aspect is broader: an institution that can conduct local studies should also be able to carry out corresponding studies for multi-institutional trials. If enough institutions are ready to carry out such studies routinely, many questions of good operation can be assessed.

Several institutions have already developed themselves into firms. Some examples are the Regenstreif Medical Center, Indianapolis; Brook Army Medical Center; Cleveland Metropolitan General Hospital; University Hospitals of Cleveland; Worcester Memorial Hospital; Henry Ford Medical Center, Detroit; Harborview Hospital, Seattle; and the St. Louis Veterans Administration.

Among the trials carried out at the Cleveland Metropolitan General Hospital [7] are studies that asked such questions as: Does feedback to resident physicians about costs of laboratory tests they order reduce the number ordered? (Yes.) Do reminders to carry out appropriate preventive procedures increase their use for ambulatory patients? (Yes.) Does a special intravenous therapy team reduce the rate of infections and complications (such as phlebitis)? (Yes, so much so that the specialized team was retained in the presence of a cost-cutting program.)

At a conference devoted to the idea of the firm [5], it became clear that it takes a long time to work out the problems of dividing hospitals into such groups—previous history obviously matters. The logistics are complicated. The nurses like the approach because it gives them fewer physicians to deal with, and it gives them more repeat patients. They get to know the patients better. Firms also seem beneficial for teaching new physicians, because the patients are often the same ones the physicians saw before, and the nurses are as well.

The idea of the firm has a great deal of promise, and its development should be accelerated.

Economic Analyses

Thus far in this chapter we have discussed the desirability of organizing information from clinical trials, of creating new trials designed in different ways, and establishing stronger follow-up for innovations. The product of these investigations would primarily be information about the safety and efficacy of various medical procedures. We need information of other kinds, too, if we are to take the costs of procedures into account. In comparing the worth of different therapies we need, among other information, the financial costs and benefits associated with diagnosis and treatment. How much has been spent on the procedures, and what costs have been saved as a result of the procedures? For instance, society benefits financially when patients recover and are able to resume work or when they can take care of themselves instead of being cared for.

Adams and her colleagues [8] reviewed the economic analyses concerning evaluations of new therapies. They found that few randomized trials had associated with them any economic analyses. It could be argued that randomized trials may not be the best occasion for making economic evaluations. But the investigators also reviewed other economic analyses of interventions and found that they were often inadequately executed. They found improper allocation of overhead costs, lack of sensitivity analyses, and few studies that aggregated treatment costs and their consequences. We need to give more attention to the quality of these appraisals if we are to improve our understanding of the financial aspects of medical procedures. In addition, we need to improve training in this component of technology assessment.

Summing up the Contributions to Quality of Life

As we've noted throughout this book, it is difficult to sum up the values of incommensurable benefits and losses. When we consider medical technologies that prolong life, we can often add up the additional time that might be gained by different therapeutic devices to calculate an approximate total expected life extension. When we need to evaluate quality of life, however, it is not easy to add up the benefits or compare them with gains in length of life.

The reader will recall that by "health-related quality of life" we refer to a person's ability to care for him- or herself, to participate in leisure-time activities, to work at an occupation, to live without pain, and to enjoy a satisfactory mental life. Thus we are discussing increasing the comfort, function, and convenience of the patient rather than saving a life.

How are we to measure an increase in comfort and convenience? We might try to make comparisons based on responses to queries like, "How many years of life would you be willing to give up to have your arthritic pain relieved for five years?" If we had answers to such questions from many people, we might create a scale of treatments and their benefits in terms of years of life. More complicated methods involving potential gambles may also be used to try to make comparisons through utility theory. Some people are skeptical about these methods because the patient does not actually make the forfeit, or because the respondents do not understand or have experience with the gambles they are asked to judge. Even responses that seem sensible and consistent may not be convincing to skeptics.

We know that some treatments relieve pain, others improve function, and others prevent disease or deterioration. When we devise a general health care system, attention must be given to the costs associated with these various contributions to quality of life. Some forms of care could be justified because they actually generate a profit for society, as when the patient is restored to the work force and contributes positively to the economy or when future health costs are reduced as a result of treatment. Many forms of care improve the patient's life but do not show such a profit. Consequently, we need ratings or orderings that help us decide which treatments we can afford.

It would be very useful to find satisfactory ways to assess gains or improvements in quality of life that can give valid and acceptable comparisons with years of life extended. Americans make five doctor's visits a year, on average. Many of these visits are to reassure ourselves that some symptom is not a harbinger of a grave disease, and usually physicians can give such assurances. What is it worth to get such anxiety-relieving diagnoses? Because improved quality of life is the primary goal of much of medicine, we very much need values for these kinds of improvements. We have some methods (Patrick and Erickson [9] give an extensive exposition of these), but they are not widely understood or accepted.

Personal Interest in Clinical Trials

What should clinical trials mean to each of us personally? If the findings from clinical trials are to apply to our personal care and that of our families, then representativeness matters. In other words, we want the trials to be carried out on people like us. If they are not, then the results will be generalized to some population rather different from our own.

Perhaps one has this selfish thought—let others take the risks by being in the experiments. This is similar to the idea that "If everyone else is vaccinated, I don't need to be." Both thoughts are dangerous not only to your health but also to your family and to people who are similar to you.

We should not think narrowly of the single clinical trial dealing with some one complaint we or our loved ones are likely to have. Rather, we should recognize that many clinical trials are being carried out and that we want their findings to be applicable to us and our families later in life. We want evidence-based medicine for ourselves. Consequently, on the rare occasions we are offered an opportunity to participate, we should probably sign up. If the trial concerns a therapy that may be changed, then the findings may ultimately be helpful to us personally, even if we did not get what turned out to be the best treatment employed in the trial. It is probably better to think of the trial as part of a system we are supporting: even if the study we participate in never affects us, we may benefit from the results of other trials for other ailments. We want the findings of these other trials to be applicable to us.

It is cheering to know that people who participate in clinical trials generally have better outcomes than people treated for the same disease who do not participate, though this advantage is partly due to the exclusion of patients with multiple diseases, at least in early trials.

Sometimes ethical arguments are raised against randomized clinical trials. By withholding a favorable new therapy, for example, the trial imposes a sacrifice on the members of the control group. Another objection is that those in the experimental group are exposed to additional risk. These arguments both seem to imply that the investigators know in advance what the trial is designed to discover. To see what happened empirically, Gilbert, McPeek, and Mosteller [10] reviewed 47 comparative studies of innovations and standard treatments in surgery and anesthesia, all they could find in that specified interval. About 49 percent of the innovations were preferred to the standard (some comparisons were regarded as equal and therefore got a score of 1/2), nearer to 50–50 than we would have expected. Since innovations brought to clinical trials are usually expected to be sure winners, this finding in the area of surgery and anesthesia that only about one-half of the new treatments were successful gives strong evidence of the value of empirical checking.

It might be argued that the patient's primary physician may have views as to which treatment is preferable. When the patient has medical contra-indications to a treatment, then of course these views should be acted upon. But aside from contraindications, the fact that responsible investigators are mounting a trial, together with the kind of empirical evidence we already have described, suggests that documentation for having a preference one way or the other is not available. In most comparisons the differences observed are likely to be small, usually less than 10 percent. Consequently, estimation is a difficult task. Our goal to improve therapies requires that we detect and retain small (and large) gains and reject therapies producing large and small losses.

When we think of the costs of clinical trials, we should be balancing them against the cost of the long-term use of therapies that are less beneficial than the proposed innovation, or perhaps even harmful. Sometimes the costs of trials are exaggerated because they include the costs of the therapies. Usually treatments will be given in any case, and so those costs should not be regarded as costs of trials. It is the marginal cost of managing patient care in the trial and recording and analyzing results that needs to be assessed.

Summary

The problems and opportunities we have considered in this chapter can lead to improvements in our capacity to evaluate new technologies, or to measure attributes of old technologies still in widespread use. The issues raised here are broader than those illustrated by any particular medical innovation, and we believe that they will retain their importance in the face of whatever reforms are to be visited upon the health sector.

Our study of these issues has led to the recommendations that follow (they are also listed in Chapter 19 with the recommendations derived from the individual case studies):

(1) Cochrane's dream of having all the clinical trials in medicine collected, organized, and, where appropriate, further synthesized is a worthy goal for medicine, and we look forward to progress through the evolving Cochrane Collaboration. Foundations, government agencies, and researchers should consider how they can best contribute to the effort.

(2) Peto's idea of simple but large clinical trials has much to recommend it, partly to decrease costs but also to increase generality.

(3) The merits of a strong post-marketing surveillance system should be carefully evaluated by the Centers for Disease Control (CDC). Any plan must recognize the substantial costs involved, especially under our current medical system, so that we can see whether long-term monitoring would likely be cost-effective.

(4) The system of firms set up to carry out trials in larger hospitals, although developing slowly, offers great potential for increasing the number of investigations of value to the institutions involved as well as to the entire health care system. The Agency for Health Care Policy and Research (AHCPR) should continue to encourage its further growth.

(5) Improved economic evaluations of treatments and programs should occur naturally, given the ever-increasing pressure on the health care

system to control costs. The evidence is that evaluations need to be improved and that we need more of them. Groups planning to carry out economic evaluations, such as cost-effectiveness analysis, should be sure to include personnel on their team with training in economics and health care financing.

(6) Although the goal of much of medicine is improved comfort and convenience rather than life-saving, we have not so far created a suitable mechanism for measuring the contributions of different treatments to quality of life in a way that makes it feasible and reasonable for consumers to compare benefits and risks of treatment. Researchers in this area should be careful to represent consumers' concerns as they develop their indices.

(7) We citizens need to appreciate our own role in the evaluation of medicine. If we do not participate in the evaluations, then our own biological idiosyncracies will not be represented in the pool of responses to the treatments. Hence the treatments found most effective may not be known to meet our personal needs.

18

Innovation-Specific Improvements

FREDERICK MOSTELLER AND HOWARD S. FRAZIER

Introduction

The United States of America has a complex health system. People over 65 years of age belong to a national health care system called Medicare, which pays for certain treatments and not others. Other citizens belong to health insurance plans arranged through their employers; certain special groups get some help from a national system called Medicaid; and the Veterans Administration offers care to current and prior members of the armed forces and their families. Still other citizens do not belong to any health plan but are able to pay for their care on a fee-for-service basis. Finally, 25 to 35 million people can neither afford to pay for needed health services nor buy health insurance that will cover their neeeds. Even though this hodgepodge arrangement has been of great concern for decades, the nation has not made a new plan. Most citizens want a universal health program for the country but as of this writing none has been implemented. Changes of such great magnitude will require lengthy political debate, and paying for them will likely be painful.

In this chapter we collect lessons learned from the case studies of Chapters 3 through 16. These lessons may be of help in improving health care whatever national health program may be adopted, because the findings seem likely to apply in almost any system that is devised. We do not address here the proposed revolution in the U.S. health care system but make suggestions, drawn from our experience in technology assessment, that may be of value in any system.

Thus, from a statistical point of view we are using the case study method to generate lessons that may be helpful to the health care system. In all we have fourteen case studies. Each deals with an important problem. We often find that a treatment for a disease or condition is not as effective—indeed, in some instances, not nearly as effective—in actual use as it could be shown to be in formal tests. This discrepancy also interests us, since it offers the possibility of improving treatment results.

From our perspective on the case studies, we see a need to focus on the following issues: (1) the penalties associated with the over-rapid introduction of new technologies into a medical system; (2) the problems found with prevention and screening technologies; (3) the advantages of patient empowerment; (4) access to care limited by problems other than money; (5) copayments and other financial barriers to health care access; and (6) behavioral changes on the part of patients and caregivers.

Rapid Diffusion of New Technologies

When totally new technologies are introduced in the United States, they create a dilemma for the medical system. Unless the technology is a drug or a device that is under the regulation of the Food and Drug Administration, the government has no authority over the use of the technology and its dissemination except insofar as it may have some control over reimbursement for delivery of the service. Even there the protection is weak, because much of demand for new products is driven by the patients. When they hear that a new treatment is available, they naturally want it for themselves, and they are unlikely to understand that the therapy may not yet have been tested or evaluated.

In 1993, for example, we saw demand overtake the assessment of medications used for patients who are HIV-positive or who have AIDS. Such patients were understandably eager to be treated with the newest medications when they first appeared and were dissatisfied with a process that rather slowly evaluates a new drug. Consequently, many were treated with these new drugs. As more information became available, in some instances it turned out that the drugs have not been beneficial but may actually have caused harm. Some patients now say that they had no idea that the medications might be harmful and blame the medical profession and the government for not protecting them.

Even in heated arguments of this sort, we should of course try to make sure that the patient has given informed consent for administration of medications not well tested. A patient with a life-threatening disease may not feel it reasonable to wait until safety has been established and would prefer to take the chance that a useful treatment has been discovered. These are very complicated matters, and those involved need our best thoughts about how both to protect them and yet give them opportunities for informed risk-taking.

An important issue concerns the overall evaluative process. When barriers to untested treatments are let down, they reduce the effectiveness of the whole process because they offer exceptions that can be used as examples. We should take care that, in the course of giving every consideration to those in life-threatening situations, we do not simultaneously destroy our mechanisms for protecting the general public. Before we had an effective Food and Drug Administration (FDA), almost any nostrum, however outrageous the claims for it, could be pressed upon the public. People who would be likely to believe unrealistic advertisements are probably present today in even larger numbers than there were before the FDA existed. And the motives for trying to sell empty promises are the same as ever. Thus our finding must be that we need to preserve our ability to protect the public.

When laparoscopy (Chapter 3) came to be used in place of open cholecystectomy, a sudden increase in the use of the method led to dangerously rapid diffusion, overwhelming the system for training surgeons. Doctors were eager to learn the new method, patients wanted it, and the educational and regulatory leadership within hospitals could not cope with the intensity of demand. Increased rates of damage to the bile ducts were overt manifestations of the hurried installation of the new operation.

Surgical regulation does not ordinarily fall under the FDA. Much of medicine does not. One lesson here is that the medical profession would do itself and the nation a service if it developed and agreed on appropriate steps to take when exciting innovations are to be disseminated to large numbers of physicians and patients.

Earlier input into the process of defining indications for the new intervention, involvement in establishing the content of training, and sponsorship of training programs are all contributions that the medical specialty societies could make. Conflicts of interest inherent in industry sponsorship of training programs can be reduced by involving the specialty societies more. Although credentialing within individual hospitals supports local accountability, more standardization seems desirable and could be promoted by the specialty societies.

Although the technical component of a service, drug, or item of equipment may be evaluated by a centralized arrangement, the essential components of skill and judgment probably are best supported and assessed at the point of delivery of the service. The goal would be to create an alliance of physician and institution, usually a hospital, for the purpose of continually evaluating performance.

When new technologies like laparoscopic cholecystectomy are introduced, extra training of the physicians is required as well as new equipment. Some of the equipment may not be reusable, and so the operation may be more expensive to carry out even though the time spent in the hospital is reduced drastically. After the innovation is introduced, training of new physicians may be conducted in medical schools, and the original costs of the equipment and their upkeep may be reduced. This evolution stimulates us to ask when it is reasonable for a new technology to be offered at reduced prices. Society needs a schedule for review of such issues.

Solutions to problems, whether they are introduced rapidly or slowly, create their own troubles. Policymakers say that last year's fix is next year's problem. For example, blood transfusions help a patient with anemia but endanger the patient with the small but real threats of hepatitis and HIV. This possibility requires that new attention be paid to the management of the blood bank. Improvement in the care of teeth among young people means that more older people will keep their own teeth for longer periods, creating a demand for more care. The sudden spread of laparoscopy for gallbladder disease temporarily led to a higher ratio of damage of bile ducts during surgery. Attempts to control the costs of the use of epoetin to treat end stage renal disease by changing reimbursement rules led providers to change their policy about treatment. The result was poorer care, at least temporarily, until the reimbursement policy was rearranged. No one would advocate making insulin unavailable, yet its effectiveness in enhancing survival of diabetics exposed the late complications of diabetic retinopathy, nerve damage, and disease of the large arteries. The unintended consequences of improvements often are not anticipated. When improvements are made, a general alert should be called to attend promptly to undesirable consequences.

The failure of one system often helps create a breakdown in another. For example, when ill health forces one to give up a job, the worker may then lose health insurance and thereby be forced to forgo care just when it is most needed. High blood pressure injures organs and over time increases the likelihood of stroke. The same kind of functional interdependence may be present in health-related institutions—in other words, systemic failures are self-perpetuating rather than self-correcting. This problem needs attention as systems in the health sector are redesigned.

When new technologies are approved for use, they often wind up costing the insurance system more than had been anticipated. Initially it may be supposed that only severe cases will be treated, for example, but, as in the case of hypertension, it may turn out that less severe cases also benefit from treatment. Then physicians will not wish to withhold the treatment. Alternative uses for a treatment often emerge, swelling the list of users. Sometimes the anticipated reductions in costs accompanying wide use are not realized. It may also happen that patients request certain treatments or diagnostic techniques so urgently that physicians give them to avoid malpractice suits rather than to provide effective therapy. So many differences from the original forecast can occur that estimates of the future cost of using a new technology cannot be taken for more than they are— guesses based on very specific assumptions that cannot be guaranteed to hold true.

Although some clinical trials are carried out in a single institution, many are organized by a consortium of institutions and have thousands of patients enrolled. Why do we have such big trials? One difficulty in medicine is that small differences in rates amount to a great deal of gain to the system as a whole. For example, around 5 percent of people aged 65 and over die each year. If we had a treatment that reduced this rate by one-half of a percent, it would represent a 10 percent reduction in the death rate for this group, an impressive effect. It takes big samples to detect an effect of this size. To get large samples of patients with a particular disease requires recruitment from many institutions, because there may be relatively few patients of a given kind in a hospital. Because practices change rather rapidly, we need to gather the data quickly for it to be relevant. In order to do that we have to pool information from many sources. Pooling has additional advantages. By spreading the inquiry over many sources of patients, we also gain diversity and thus generality of findings. Put another way, the necessity for speed also forces us to fulfill the requirement of diversity.

Prevention and Screening

The opportunities to help society on a large scale at relatively low cost per person make preventive methods particularly attractive. Among the cases we have studied, vaccines (Chapter 9), fluoride in dentistry (Chapter 12), screening for hypertension (Chapter 10), screening for visual handicaps (Chapter 11), and continuation therapy for the recovered depressive (Chapter 5) have each provided some lessons.

In the case of vaccines, the first lesson is that a disease that is not wiped out is likely to rebound even when we seem to have it in control. Measles is just such a disease. After the number of cases dropped from 450,000 in 1964 to a little over 6,000 in 1986, the incidence of measles began to increase. The success of measles vaccine was impressive, but the public does not have a clear conviction that measles is a serious disease or that immunization is valuable. People have not been persuaded to demand vaccines. Why has appropriate immunization not been delivered in timely fashion?For one thing, apparently no one is accountable for making sure that vaccines have been delivered to the patient: not the doctor, not the patient nor the patient's parent, not the local public health department.

We have no effective personal health surveillance system. Individuals do not have a lifetime booklet of their health experience, as individuals in some countries have, that tells what diseases and treatments they have experienced. When the patient has a personal physician, a record of this kind is kept, at least of those matters that the personal physician handles.

Some of the barriers to vaccination that have been found when professionals inquire why children have not been vaccinated include rules requiring that one must have a pre-existing appointment to be vaccinated, or a required physical examination before vaccination, or prior enrollment in a health system, or be prepared to pay administrative fees. When one looks at the history of children who have not been vaccinated at appropriate times, one finds that there usually have been many previous opportunities to vaccinate the child. One solution that would help would be to vaccinate a child at the site where it has been recognized that a vaccination has been omitted. Another desirable change would be to make certain that insurers will reimburse for immunization.

Fluoridation seems to have been a big success. It has improved the teeth of millions with none of the hazards that many had predicted. Adding fluoride to the public water supply is, of course, a "Big Brother" sort of policy, of a kind that we cannot often expect to have available. Fluoride is easily distributed at low cost to the whole population. The objections to its use seem to involve issues of civil liberty—the fact that the majority can tyrannize the minority by taking steps of which the minority disapproves.

Originally, hypertension was not considered a disease, but once its hazards were understood and some useful treatments were available, screening for hypertension became a valuable tool. Through multipronged educational, screening, and treatment programs, members of minority groups needing treatment are apparently being treated relatively more frequently than hypertensive individuals among the majority. This seems to mean that when appropriately designed educational programs call sufficiently forcefully upon the attention of minority groups, they will respond effectively. We should study the success of the antihypertension program in reaching the minority sufferers. This relative success is especially noteworthy because the patient does not ordinarily have symptoms that would suggest an illness. Perhaps this success can be reproduced for other diseases.

The need for screening is evident for another common problem—loss of visual acuity. As is true of hypertension, people do not ordinarily recognize for themselves that they are losing acuity, even though they may say that they have to hold a newspaper further and further away from their eyes to read it. The lesson again is that regular screening is valuable if the patient is to make the most of life.

An important finding emphasized by the cases on hypertension, diabetic retinopathy, and eye injury is that government, industry, the medical profession, and society can, over a period of time, identify individuals at risk from a disease and find ways to diminish its impact. The work on hypertension, for example, was carried on by large numbers from each interest group, and after some decades outstanding progress was made. As another example, the routine use of screening surveys for depression offers a valid, inexpensive way to detect new cases of the disease.

The Therapeutic Alliance

In theory, at least, the right of the competent patient to accept or refuse preferred treatment is widely acknowledged, although decisions other than acceptance are in general not encouraged. Now we are learning that definite advantage accrues when the patient is invited into a therapeutic alliance with the caregiver. The advantages of allowing the patient to take an active role in treatment were explored in the case of patient-controlled analgesia in Chapter 8. Within safe limits of dosage, control by the postoperative patient of the administration of pain-relieving drugs results in greater patient satisfaction, better control of pain, and no greater use of medication than standard therapy. Furthermore, preoperative teaching about the surgical experience and relaxation techniques resulted in lower usage of opiates and shorter hospital stays.

The overall lessons seem to be, first, that it is advantageous to the patient to be informed and to be enlisted as an active, decision-making participant in the therapeutic process. Second, it seems prudent to seek and test additional ways of empowering patients in the interests of improving outcomes of treatment, even though monitoring by trained personnel still will be necessary.

Access to Health Care

Although we often think that the only barrier to access to health care is financial, primarily owing to lack of membership in some version of our insurance system, other barriers we have been discussing are important as well. For example, although several effective treatments are available for unipolar depression (Chapter 5), they are used only about half as often as they should be. Some reasons are that people with this disease tend to avoid others, and even sufferers examined by a physician may not be properly diagnosed, presumably because of inadequate training of the physician. Thus two possibilities for improvement suggest themselves. The straightforward one is that teaching hospitals need to be made aware of the high rate of misdiagnosis of this disease (and as a generalization, no doubt, other diseases also, such as diabetic retinopathy) and to take steps to change the training in these aggravated instances. A second possibility is more delicate. Is it appropriate to invade the privacy of people who do not seem to want to have any interaction with others, with the intent of discovering whether they need medical care and then delivering it? This sort of intervention needs broad discussion and the development of some consensus within a culture before widespread use.

In the field of organ transplantation (Chapter 6), we have found a number of barriers to access. First, better genetic matching of donors and recipients of organs is needed to increase the probability that transplantation succeeds. Second, in our society many fewer donor organs are available than could profitably be used. The reasons are multiple, some having to do with personal or religious beliefs, some with misunderstandings about the process and the need, and some having to do with problems of size. It is more difficult to find genetic matches in smaller than in larger subgroups. Thus minority groups may suffer reduced access to transplanted organs not only because the pool of donors is smaller but also because a smaller percentage of the group offers to donate. The simple step that probably would do most to make additional organs available would be to introduce a policy of "presumed consent," essentially the opposite of what the current legal situation in the United States holds.

Unless a person has actively shown a willingness to donate his or her organs, the law usually presumes that the organs are not available for transplanting. In some countries the opposite is held—that unless opposition to the use of the organs has been expressed, consent to such use is presumed. Obviously, such a complete turnaround in the legal position requires consideration and discussion, and we encourage such a movement. As far as we know, no one suggests that organs be used if a person has expressed specific opposition to being a donor.

In some states, institutions are required, in the event of a person's death, to ask the surviving family members whether they wish to donate organs for transplantation. Although there is evidence that many families are somewhat comforted by having the opportunity to allow organ donations, many institutions do not seem to carry out the initial request. Perhaps some unhappy experiences have led them to omit this duty. Proposing donorship needs to be encouraged.

At present in the United States, it is illegal to traffic in organs—to sell or buy them. At the moment there seems to be no pressing reason to try to change this position; changing it would open up serious possibilities of abuse that might be very difficult to control.

Although we have reviewed only kidney transplants, other organs are subject to much the same issues, the exception being that people have two kidneys and seem to be able to survive well with only one. Consequently, the possibility of a living donor giving up one kidney, especially to a close relative in need, is available, whereas other organs may not be donated under the same conditions.

For a health care system to get high marks, several dimensions need to be considered. For example, within reason we want persons suffering from a disease to be found, diagnosed, and treated. When technologies are being distributed, especially expensive ones, the system must strive for fairness. When treatment is delivered to members of different groups at different rates—as seems to be the case for individuals with hypertension, or those who require total joint replacement or organ transplantation—questions of equity arise. Consequently, organizations that are responsible for distributing treatments do well to examine the rates of use by various groups and to consider whether any disparities need attention. Obviously, enormous numbers of groups could be considered, but a standard demographic set that can be routinely examined are age, gender, ethnic group, and socioeconomic status. Such investigations require considerable sensitivity to medical as well as social problems. Even if disparities in rates occur, they may be well grounded in empirical experience. For example, if people over 85 years old are rarely being given certain operations even though they have symptoms suggesting that they are appropriate candidates, it may be that experience shows such patients have a low survival rate following the operations. The point is that monitoring the distribution of care will help avoid both favoritism and neglect, as well as provide information about how the process of allocation of resources is working.

Copayments and Reimbursements

Problems of cost and reimbursement affect access to care. Although Medicare will pay 80 percent of the cost of hip and knee replacement, the total costs of such operations including rehabilitation can be very high. Thus, for every $10,000 of total cost, the patient would be required to supply $2,000. For a $50,000 operation, the patient would be responsible for $10,000. These operations are usually done in older people, who ordinarily will not have the income to cover high copayments.

Some argue that, on the basis of economic analysis, it is not clear that society will benefit from reduced costs of future health care by investing in operations for the elderly. The "future savings" argument for delivering services—that care delivered today may prevent the need for costlier care later—does not apply to the elderly as it does to the young. In some instances, therefore, people will not have access to treatment under our system, even though they may need the operation to take care of their everyday living needs. The question is whether society regards these expensive operations as treatments that ought to be delivered even when re-entry into the work force is not an issue. The main purpose of the operation is to improve quality of life by reducing pain and improving mobility. Such gains, rather than return to the workplace, would be the justification for giving the operation to an older person. This needs national discussion.

Similarly, we have seen in Chapter 7 that a patient using epoetin for treatment of anemia in end stage renal disease needs to take the medicine regularly for a lifetime, unless a transplant becomes available. Again, the patient is required to pay 20 percent of the total cost of an expensive medication. Do we want to deny the patient this treatment if the financing is not available? It seems more appropriate to set the reimbursement policies to accomplish the medical goals of treatment. Society needs to spend more time thinking about what treatments it is willing to give to those who have medical needs. Some studies of this matter have been made (especially in Oregon, which is experimenting with setting priorities for treating diseases within a budget), but so far the results have been confusing. Enforced rationing in a universal health care system will require us to consider carefully what treatments are to be made universally available. Some states, including Oregon, are going to introduce new systems for universal health care, and their experience may help us with these choices [1].

A transplant patient must take expensive medication for years to prevent the immunologic rejection of the new organ. Under current health care arrangements, this medication is paid for by the health system for the first year, but after that the payment shifts to the patient. Ordinarily the patient will not be in much better position to pay for the medication after a year than he or she was before. Without the medication, the transplant is very likely to fail. Our society needs to think through our attitude toward various charges.

As we have mentioned earlier, the fragmentation of sources of financial support for health services and of responsibility for their delivery is a prominent feature of the health sector in the United States. The existence of multiple budgets and divided responsibility tends to conceal the advantages of many services and to obscure the injurious effects of the system. One example is immunization against measles. Put aside for the moment the tragic reduction in quality of life of children who become retarded or deaf as a result of preventable episodes of measles. In our system, the dollar costs of a more aggressive program of immunization fall on one set of societal agents, while the financial effects of preventing—or failing to prevent—deafness and mental retardation are borne by other social institutions supported by other financial sources. Another example is joint replacement for the treatment of severely symptomatic degenerative arthritis. This expensive but effective operation may change the patient's status from total disability, requiring bed and chair care with nursing support, to one of self-care. Our present way of handling the financial consequences of the decisions about an individual patient's care effectively prevents us from understanding the overall financial consequences of the system's management of the illness.

The existence of multiple budgets and multiple agents attenuates the connection between cause and effect, responsibility and accountability. This mode of organization increases the real cost of effective health services while inhibiting their distribution, and it encourages cost-shifting among providers, payers, and patients. We do not have the opportunity for more detailed examination of this problem here, but we urge our readers to bear it in mind as an important influence on the societal benefits that can be realized from potentially successful innovations.

Improving Outcomes through Behavioral Changes in Patients and Caregivers

To be successful, medical innovations require modifications in the behavior of those who use the health services delivery system to give or receive care. The cases described in the previous chapters illustrate the variety of behavioral changes that must accompany an innovation. Although the behavioral changes may arise in many different ways, typically they originate as the result of training. We illustrate here the pervasiveness of this need for training.

First, we call attention to the performance of the caregivers. If society is to benefit from the greatly improved treatments for depression or for diabetic retinopathy, for example, an important step is training primary-care practitioners to use available screening instruments and to refer their patients for further evaluation. In the case of control of perioperative pain, education is needed to foster recognition by caregivers of the advantages of better pain control and the inadequacies of conventional treatment and to validate the shift of responsibility for administering pain medication to the patient.

Second, we mention the positive effects of patient empowerment, with respect not only to administration of pain-relieving medications as described above but also to an improved understanding by the patient of the course of the treatment process.

Third, as we note in the case of laparoscopy and anesthesiology, organized medicine, through its specialty societies, is able to encourage standard setting and describe indications and hazards of innovative treatments. The specialty societies are in a particularly advantageous position to sponsor and direct training programs in the appropriate use of the new technology.

Fourth, for some innovations, successful implementation requires complex, multipronged programs of administration. Without these carefully crafted applications, the innovation achieves only a fraction of its potential. We offer as examples the cases on immunization and the detection and control of hypertension. We suggest that success in these areas can be improved by seeking the experience and suggestions of experts in public health.

Fifth, and finally, we need to create a culture of understanding and support for rigorous technology assessment. This will require of all participants in the design, delivery, and use of health services a receptivity to the lessons that can be taught by statisticians and epidemiologists.

Summary

The fourteen cases we have described in this book support a fundamental conclusion: in order to enhance the benefits of medical innovations, reduce risks from their use, and conserve resources, rigorous evaluation by standard methods is essential. Because the adoption of any medical innovation requires the commitment of resources, it usually involves decisions about policy. These decisions are powerfully informed by technology assessment and by systematic efforts to discover the preferences for various medical services on the part of our fellow citizens.

Our purpose in writing this book is to influence the methods we use in making certain kinds of decisions. In support of this orientation to action, we include here recommendations derived from the cases.

(1) Good scientists and good science and medicine do not assure the invention of good therapies, and so any therapy ought to be proved safe and effective by a recognized agency using standard criteria before its introduction to the general public. Drugs and some devices must be approved by the Food and Drug Administration (FDA), but other forms of treatment, like surgery, are not subject to approval. The Executive and Congress should plan a decade-long revision that would bring these other kinds of treatments under the tent of the FDA.

(2) When technologies of higher cost are only modestly more beneficial than less expensive ones, guidelines for treatment issued by specialist societies and under the aegis of government agencies may recommend first trying the less expensive ones and using the more expensive ones only when the initial treatment fails.

(3) To reduce overhead costs in the health sector, the Health Care Financing Administration (HCFA) and other payers should consider two administrative changes:

(3a) Develop a universal system of simplified billing and bookkeeping;

(3b) Enhance control over malpractice while compensating injured patients more fairly and reliably than does the present tort system.

(4) The rapid introduction of a new technology may on occasion strain the medical education and credentialing systems and lead to temporary additional mortality and morbidity in patients. Under these circumstances, the specialty societies should assume leadership in formulating indications and standards. It is important that the urgency of the problem not prevent the protection of the public.

(5) New methods may at first be more expensive than previous treatments, for a variety of understandable reasons. A procedure for considering appropriate intervals for reviewing prices would be helpful. The Executive should ask the HCFA to review this matter and give advice, and Congress should ask the General Accounting Office (GAO) to make corresponding inquiries and suggestions.

(6) A system is needed for tracking immunization, at least in children, and this should include a plan for performing the immunization wherever it is found that immunization has been omitted.

(7) Multifaceted educational and screening programs such as those for hypertension should be established to promote other health care services, such as vaccination.

(8) In the field of organ transplantation, a most important step would be to discuss changing the national policy to that of "presumed consent." A national discussion of this matter sponsored by the HCFA and the ESRD program would probably lead either to a change in policy, initiated through the Congress, or at least to many more volunteer donors.

(9) The current arrangements for payments and copayments for various treatments seem often to be internally inconsistent and counterproductive. A new health program sponsored by the Congress and carried out by the Institute of Medicine should review the payment system with these problems in mind.

(10) If we are to have a national health care system, the wishes of the public concerning the delivery of health services must be made clear. Experimental programs by the states may help us reach some consensus by exploring the preferences people show for allocation of health care resources.

(11) In order to deliver the benefits of greatly improved treatments for depression or for diabetic retinopathy, for example, teaching hospitals, medical schools, and specialty societies need to train primary-care practitioners to use available screening instruments and to refer their patients for further evaluation.

(12) Modern methods of handling pain must be made known both to patients and caregivers, as effective pain relief is needed to speed recovery of patients after surgery and to improve the quality of life of the patient with chronic pain. Departments of surgery and anesthesia should take leadership in disseminating the information about modern practice, and hospitals should install quality-control procedures to assure that the most appropriate methods are actually used. Both the National Institutes of Health and the Agency for Health Care Policy and Research plan to support studies related to such dissemination and practice.

(13) News of the benefits of patient empowerment—that educating the patient about the course of treatment and recovery improves the rate of recovery, and that allowing patients to administer their own pain-relieving medications enhances the effect of the drugs—should be disseminated to caregivers. Patients should be encouraged to appreciate their own role in recovering from illnesses.

For convenience, we repeat in Chapter 19 all the recommendations from Chapters 17 and 18.

19

Recommendations for Change

HOWARD S. FRAZIER AND FREDERICK MOSTELLER

Introduction

Anyone making practical recommendations for large heterogeneous societies should do so with caution. In a few instances a fairly clear mandate
for change can be devised, because little opposition is anticipated or
because no other approach is likely to achieve the goal. But in the usual
situation matters are more complicated, and few people are fully aware of
the details of the current system or the benefits and risks of possible
alternatives. The state of the health care system in the United States is
certainly one of the "more complicated" matters.

When complex problems confront a democratic society, initial discussion may be more valuable than a clear but controversial and sudden
decision. Although unanimity may not be reached through discussion,
different groups may find a variety of solutions satisfactory to them and,
if these are enacted, health care may be improved as a whole even if in a
heterogeneous manner. In this spirit we offer selected actions that the
United States might undertake to improve its health care system, whatever
directions the political and economic winds may blow.

Recommendations

The first set of suggestions, discussed more fully in Chapter 17, addresses
general concerns about the quality of health care. Each recommendation
is designed to strengthen technology assessment, is under development, is
independent of particular technologies presented for evaluation, and is
independent of the details of organization of the health sector.

Organize results of clinical trials. Cochrane's dream of having all the clinical trials in medicine collected, organized, and, where appropriate, further synthesized is a worthy goal for medicine, and we look forward to progress through the evolving Cochrane Collaboration. Foundations, government agencies, and researchers should consider how they can best contribute to the effort.

Conduct more and simpler clinical trials. Peto's idea of simple but large clinical trials has much to recommend it, partly to decrease costs but also to increase generality.

Encourage more effective post-marketing surveillance. The merits of a strong post-marketing surveillance system should be carefully evaluated by the Centers for Disease Control (CDC). Any plan must recognize the substantial costs involved, especially under our current medical system, so that we can see whether long-term monitoring would likely be cost-effective.

Develop and utilize the "firm system" in our larger hospitals. The system of firms set up to carry out trials in larger hospitals, although developing slowly, offers great potential for increasing the number of investigations of value to the institutions involved as well as to the entire health care system. The Agency for Health Care Policy and Research (AHCPR) should continue to encourage its further growth.

Design better economic evaluations. Improved economic evaluations of treatments and programs should occur naturally, given the ever-increasing pressure on the health care system to control costs. The evidence is that evaluations need to be improved and that we need more of them. Groups planning to carry out economic evaluations, such as cost-effectiveness analysis, should be sure to include personnel on their team with training in economics and health care financing.

Focus on measuring quality of life. Although the goal of much of medicine is improved comfort and convenience rather than life-saving, we have not so far created a suitable mechanism for measuring the contributions of different treatments to quality of life in a way that makes it feasible and reasonable for consumers to compare benefits and risks of treatment. Researchers in this area should be careful to represent consumers' concerns as they develop their indices.

All of us should be represented in the results of clinical trials. We citizens need to appreciate our own role in the evaluation of medicine. If we do not participate in the evaluations, then our own biological idiosyncracies will not be represented in the pool of responses to the treatments. Hence the treatments found most effective may not be known to meet our personal needs.

The second group of recommendations emerges from our case studies of individual innovations whose performance seems positive and well established. These are discussed more fully in Chapter 18.

Treatments for people ultimately must be tested in people. Good scientists and good science and medicine do not assure the invention of good therapies, and so any therapy ought to be proved safe and effective by a recognized agency using standard criteria before its introduction to the general public. Conversely, the demonstration that a treatment is ineffective or harmful should be publicized to the medical profession and potential recipients to hasten its abandonment. Drugs and some devices must be approved by the Food and Drug Administration (FDA), but other forms of treatment, like surgery, are not subject to approval. The Executive and Congress should plan a decade-long revision that would bring these other kinds of treatments under the tent of the FDA.

From society's perspective, the best treatment is not always the most effective one. When technologies of higher cost are only modestly more beneficial than less expensive ones, guidelines for treatment issued by specialist societies and under the aegis of government agencies may recommend first trying the less expensive ones and using the more expensive ones only when the initial treatment fails.

Decrease overhead costs in the health care system. To reduce overhead costs in the health sector, the Health Care Financing Administration (HCFA) and other payers should consider two administrative changes: develop a universal system of simplified billing and bookkeeping; and enhance control over malpractice while compensating injured patients more fairly and reliably than does the present tort system.

The introduction of new technology should be accompanied by oversight procedures. The rapid introduction of a new technology may on occasion strain the medical education and credentialing systems and lead to temporary additional mortality and morbidity in patients. Under these circumstances, the specialty societies should assume leadership in formulating indications and standards. It is important that the urgency of the problem not prevent the protection of the public.

Widespread adoption of new methods should be followed by review of their prices. New methods may at first be more expensive than previous treatments, for a variety of understandable reasons. A procedure for considering appropriate intervals for reviewing prices would be helpful. The Executive should ask the HCFA to review this matter and give advice, and Congress should ask the General Accounting Office (GAO) to make corresponding inquiries and describe options.

Immunization in children, including development of permanent, portable immunization records, needs high priority. A system is needed for tracking immunization, at least in children, and this should include a plan for performing the immunization wherever it is found that immunization has been omitted. In addition to increasing the rate of timely immunization, the program should include a permanent, portable immunization record that stays with the child. Responsibility for planning and implementation of the program of immunization might well be given to the Centers for Disease Control.

Vaccination programs can profit from lessons learned in multifaceted screening programs for hypertension. Multifaceted educational and screening programs such as those for hypertension should be established to promote other health care services, such as vaccination.

Improved access to organ transplantation would follow from a policy of presumed consent to donation. In the field of organ transplantation, a most important step would be to discuss changing the national policy to that of "presumed consent." A national discussion of this matter sponsored by the HCFA and the ESRD program would probably lead either to a change in policy, initiated through the Congress, or at least to many more volunteer donors.

Current reimbursement policies should be reviewed to discover and eliminate perverse incentives. The current arrangements for payments and co-payments for various treatments seem often to be internally inconsistent and counterproductive. A new health program sponsored by the Congress and carried out by the Institute of Medicine should review the payment system with these problems in mind. Fragmentation of responsibility for the provision of medical services often means that services are not provided even though providing them would be cost-effective.

State-sponsored experiments in delivery of health services should be encouraged. If we are to have a national health care system, the wishes of the public concerning the delivery of health services must be made clear. Experimental programs by the states may help us reach some consensus by exploring the preferences people show for allocation of health care resources.

Training of primary practitioners should emphasize the use of screening instruments and appropriate referrals for common, serious, and treatable conditions such as diabetic retinopathy and depression. In order to deliver the benefits of greatly improved treatments for depression or for diabetic retinopathy, for example, teaching hospitals, medical schools, and specialty societies need to train primary-care practitioners to use available screening instruments and to refer their patients for further evaluation and treatment.

New techniques for controlling pain deserve wider dissemination and understanding. Modern methods of handling pain must be made known both to patients and caregivers, as effective pain relief is needed to speed recovery of patients after surgery and to improve the quality of life of the patient with chronic pain. Departments of surgery and anesthesia should take leadership in disseminating the information about modern practice, and hospitals should install quality-control procedures to assure that the most appropriate methods are actually used. Both the National Institutes of Health and the Agency for Health Care Policy and Research plan to support studies related to such dissemination and practice.

News of the benefits of patient empowerment—that educating the patient about the course of treatment and recovery improves the rate of recovery, and that allowing patients to administer their own pain-relieving medications enhances the effect of the drugs—should be disseminated to caregivers. Patients should be encouraged to appreciate their own role in recovering from illnesses.

Our case studies include many examples of effective treatment for important medical problems. These treatments often fail to live up to the potential indicated by formal evaluation. The recommendations listed above, several of which are directed to specific groups, are intended to help us achieve the full potential of medicine.

Sometimes we ask that certain groups take responsibility for specific problems, as when we suggested that medical groups be asked to attend to the hazards of new technologies implemented too rapidly. In other circumstances we propose that individuals need to examine their own roles as patients or as participants in clinical trials. In several instances, we ask researchers to help the system by creating improvements in methods of evaluation. For example, the problem of assessing the value of improvements in quality of life needs further attention if the nation is to design a health care system that will be perceived as fair.

We propose, in addition, a number of concrete steps that might improve the total performance of the system but that do not seem to depend much on how the health care system may be revised over the next few years.

The approach used here is not at all exhaustive: many more examples of effective treatments are available, and studying them no doubt would give us additional suggestions for improvements in our system. And, of course, examining treatments that seem not to be effective might offer another source of education and recommendations. The choice between these two approaches is less important than the strength of our commitment to rigorous measurement of the outcomes of medical interventions. Only by his means will we be able to identify the components of medical care worth paying for.

References

2. Evaluating Medical Technologies

1. Goldstein, P. A., Sacks, H. S., and Chalmers, T. C. 1989. Hormone administration for the maintenance of pregnancy. In Chalmers, I., Enkin, M., and Keirse, M. J. N. C. (eds.), *Effective Care in Pregnancy and Childbirth*, 612–623. Oxford: Oxford University Press.
2. Herbst, A. L., Ulfelder, H., and Poskanzer, D. C. 1971. Association of maternal stilbestrol therapy with tumor appearance in young women. *New England Journal of Medicine* 284:878–881.
3. Beecher, H. K. 1955. The powerful placebo. *Journal of the American Medical Association* 159:1602–1606.
4. Barsamian, E. M. 1977. The rise and fall of internal mammary artery ligation in the treatment of angina pectoris and the lessons learned. Chapter 13 in Bunker, J. P., Barnes, B. A., and Mosteller, F. (eds.), *Costs, Risks, and Benefits of Surgery*, 212–220. New York: Oxford University Press.
5. Cobb, L. A., et al. 1959. An evaluation of internal-mammary-artery ligation by a double-blind technique. *New England Journal of Medicine* 260:1115–1118.
6. Dimond, E. G., Kittle, C. F., and Crockett, J. E. 1958. Evaluation of internal mammary artery ligation and sham procedure in angina pectoris. *Circulation* 18:712–713.
7. Fowler, F. J., Jr., et al. 1988. Symptom status and quality of life following prostatectomy. *Journal of the American Medical Association* 259:3018–3022.
8. Fowler, F. J., Jr., et al. 1993. Patient-reported complications and follow-up treatment after radical prostatectomy: The national Medicare experience: 1988–1990 (updated June 1993). *Urology* 42:622–629.
9. Fuchs, V. R. 1974. *Who Shall Live? Health, Economics, and Social Choice.* New York: Basic Books.
10. Chalmers, I., Enkin, M., and Keirse, M. J. N. C. (eds.). 1989. *Effective Care in Pregnancy and Childbirth.* Oxford: Oxford University Press.

11. Committee for Evaluating Medical Technologies in Clinical Use. 1985. *Assessing Medical Technologies.* Council on Health Care Technology, Institute of Medicine. Washington, D.C.: National Academy Press.
12. Goodman, C. (ed.). 1988. *Medical Technology Assessment Directory.* Council on Health Care Technology, Institute of Medicine. Washington, D.C.: National Academy Press.
13. Emanuel, E. J., and Emanuel, L. L. 1994. The economics of dying: The illusion of cost-savings at the end of life. *New England Journal of Medicine* 330:540–544.
14. Grimes, D. A. 1993. Technology follies: The uncritical acceptance of medical innovation. *Journal of the American Medical Association* 269:3030–3033.
15. Angell, M. 1993. How much will health care reform cost? *New England Journal of Medicine* 328:1778–1779.
16. Gittelsohn, A. M., and Wennberg, J. E. 1977. On the incidence of tonsillectomy and other common surgical procedures. Chapter 7 in Bunker, J. P., Barnes, B. A., and Mosteller, F. (eds.), *Costs, Risks, and Benefits of Surgery,* 91–106. New York: Oxford University Press.
17. Patrick, D. L., and Erickson, P. 1993. *Health Status and Health Policy: Quality of Life in Health Care Evaluation and Resource Allocation.* New York: Oxford University Press.

3. Laparoscopic Cholecystectomy for Gallstones

1. Ransohoff, D. F., and Gracie, W. A. 1990. Management of patients with symptomatic gallstones: A quantitative analysis. *Americal Journal of Medicine* 88:154–160.
2. Ganey, J. B., et al. 1986. Cholecystectomy: Clinical experience with a large series. *American Journal of Surgery* 151:352–356.
3. Gilliland, T. M., and Traverso, L. W. 1990. Modern standards for comparison of cholelithiasis with emphasis on long term relief of symptoms. *Surgery, Gynecology, & Obstetrics* 170:39–44.
4. Habib, M. A., et al. 1990. Complications of cholecystectomy in district general hospitals. *British Journal of Clinical Practice* 44:189–192.
5. Herzog, U., et al. 1992. Surgical treatment for cholelithiasis. *Surgery, Gynecology, & Obstetrics* 175:238–242.
6. McSherry, C. K. 1989. Cholecystectomy: The gold standard. *American Journal of Surgery* 158:174–178.
7. Cheslyn-Curtis, S., and Russell, R. C. G. 1991. New trends in gallstone management. *British Journal of Surgery* 78:143–149.
8. *New York Times,* Aug. 14, 1990. Section C, 1:1.
9. Hoofnagle, J. H. 1992. *Introduction to the Consensus Development Conference on Gallstones and Laparoscopic Cholecystectomy.* NIH Consensus Development Conference. Bethesda: National Institutes of Health.
10. Hawasli, A., and Lloyd, L. R. 1991. Laparoscopic cholecystectomy: The learning curve: Report of 50 patients. *American Surgeon* 57:542–544.

11. Meyers, W. C. 1991. Southern surgeons club: A prospective analysis of 1518 laparoscopic cholecystectomies. *New England Journal of Medicine* 324:1073–1078.

12. Soper, N. J., et al. 1992. Laparoscopic cholecystectomy, the new "gold standard." *Archives of Surgery* 127:917–921.

13. Bailey, R. W., et al. 1991. Laparoscopic cholecystectomy, experience with 375 consecutive patients. *Annals of Surgery* 214:531–540.

14. Graves, H. A., Ballinger, J. F., and Anderson, W. J. 1991. Appraisal of laparoscopic cholecystectomy. *Annals of Surgery* 213:655–662.

15. Wittgen, C. M., et al. 1991. Analysis of the hemodynamic and ventilatory effects of laparoscopic cholecystectomy. *Archives of Surgery* 126:997–1000.

16. Jordan, A. M. 1991. Hospital charges for laparoscopic and open cholecystectomy. *Journal of the American Medical Association* 266:3425–3426.

17. Voyless, C. R., et al. 1991. A practical approach to laparoscopic cholecystectomy. *American Journal of Surgery* 161:365–370.

4. Preserving Vision in Diabetic Retinopathy

1. Davis, M. D. 1975. Proliferative diabetic retinopathy. In Ryan, S. J. (ed.), *The Retina*. Philadelphia: J. B. Lippincott.

2. Ederer, F., and Hiller, R. 1975. Clinical trials, diabetic retinopathy, and photocoagulation: A reanalysis of five studies. *Survey of Ophthalmology* 19:267–286.

3. DRS Coordinating Center. 1973. *The Diabetic Retinopathy Study: A Nationwide Clinical Trial*. Baltimore: DRS Coordinating Center.

4. Aiello, L. M., et al. 1973. The Diabetic Retinopathy Study. *Archives of Ophthalmology* 90:347–348.

5. Diabetic Retinopathy Study Research Group. 1981. Photocoagulation treatment of proliferative diabetic retinopathy: Clinical application of diabetic retinopathy study (DRS) findings. DRS Report No. 8. *Ophthalmology* 88:583–600.

6. Diabetic Retinopathy Study Research Group. 1976. *Results from the Diabetic Retinopathy Study: An Explanation for Patients*. Washington, D.C.: U.S. Department of Health, Education, and Welfare.

7. Early Treatment of Diabetic Retinopathy Study Research Group. 1991. Results from the Early Treatment of Diabetic Retinopathy Study. *Ophthalmology* 98:739–840.

8. Drummond, M. F., Davies, L. M., and Ferris, F. L., III. 1992. Assessing the costs and benefits of medical research: The Diabetic Retinopathy Study. *Social Science and Medicine* 34:973–981.

9. Javitt, J. C., et al. 1990. Detecting and treating retinopathy in patients with type I diabetes mellitus: A health policy model. *Ophthalmology* 97:483–495.

5. The Treatment of Unipolar Depression

1. Styron, W. 1990. *Darkness Visible: A Memoir of Madness*. New York: Random House.

2. Wells, K. B., et al. 1989. The functioning and well-being of depressed patients: Results from the medical outcomes study. *Journal of the American Medical Association* 262:914–919.

3. Boyd, J. H., and Weissman, M. M. 1981. Epidemiology of affective disorders: A reexamination and future directions. *Archives of General Psychiatry* 38:1039–1046.

4. Weissman, M. M., and Myers, J. K. 1978. Affective disorders in a U.S. urban community: The use of Research Diagnostic Criteria in an epidemiologic survey. *Archives of General Psychiatry* 35:1304–1311.

5. U.S. Bureau of the Census. 1991. *Statistical Abstract of the United States,* 111th edition. Washington, D.C.: U.S. Department of Commerce.

6. American Psychiatric Association. 1987. *Diagnostic and Statistical Manual of Mental Disorders,* 3rd edition. Washington, D.C.: American Psychiatric Association.

7. Belsher, G., and Costello, C. G. 1988. Relapse after recovery from unipolar depression: A critical review. *Psychological Bulletin* 104:84–96.

8. Keller, M. B., et al. 1983. Predictors of relapse in major depressive disorder. *Journal of the American Medical Association* 250:3299–3309.

9. National Center for Health Statistics. 1991. *Vital Statistics of the United States, 1988, Volume II, Mortality, Part B.* Hyattsville, MD: National Center for Health Statistics, Public Health Service.

10. Pokorny, A. D. 1964. Suicide rates in various psychiatric disorders. *Journal of Nervous and Mental Disease* 139:499–506.

11. Winokur, G., and Tsuang, M. 1975. The Iowa 500: Suicide in mania, depression and schizophrenia. *American Journal of Psychiatry* 132:650–651.

12. Leaf, P. J., et al. 1985. Contact with health professionals for the treatment of psychiatric and emotional problems. *Medical Care* 23:1322–1337.

13. Keller, M. B., et al. 1986. The persistent risk of chronicity in recurrent episodes of nonbipolar major depressive disorder: A prospective follow-up. *American Journal of Psychiatry* 143:24–28.

14. Keller, M. B., et al. 1984. Long-term outcome of episodes of major depression: Clinical and public health significance. *Journal of the American Medical Association* 252:788–792.

15. Gonzalez, L. R., Lewinsohn, P. M., and Clarke, G. N. 1985. Longitudinal follow-up of unipolar depressives: An investigation of predictors of relapse. *Journal of Consulting and Clinical Psychology* 53:461–469.

16. Lavori, P. W., Keller, M. B., and Klerman, G. L. 1984. Relapse in affective disorders: A reanalysis of the literature using life table methods. *Journal of Psychiatric Research* 18:13–25.

17. Janicak, P. G., et al. 1985. Effect of ECT: A meta-analysis. *American Journal of Psychiatry* 142:297–302.

18. Medical Research Council. 1965. Clinical trial of the treatment of depressive illness. *British Medical Journal* 1:881–886.

19. Beck, A. T. 1976. *Cognitive Therapy and the Emotional Disorders.* New York: International Universities Press.

20. Dobson, K. S. 1989. A meta-analysis of the efficacy of cognitive therapy for depression. *Journal of Consulting and Clinical Psychology* 57:414–419.
21. Steinbrueck, S. M., Maxwell, S. E., and Howard, G. S. 1983. A meta-analysis of psychotherapy and drug therapy in the treatment of unipolar depression with adults. *Journal of Consulting and Clinical Psychology* 51:856–863.
22. Prien, R. F., et al. 1984. Drug therapy in the prevention of recurrences in unipolar and bipolar affective disorders: Report of the NIMH Collaborative Study Group comparing lithium carbonate, imipramine, and a lithium carbonate–imipramine combination. *Archives of General Psychiatry* 41:1096–1104.
23. Blackburn, I. M., Eunson, K. M., and Bishop, S. 1986. A two-year naturalistic follow-up of depressed patients treated with cognitive therapy, pharmacotherapy and a combination of both. *Journal of Affective Disorders* 10:67–75.
24. Neville, D., and Weinstein, M. C. 1989. Lifetime costs and health consequences of an incident case of major depressive disorder. Unpublished manuscript.
25. Neville, D. 1989. Program evaluation: An illustration of three quantitative approaches in the field of health promotion. From a dissertation completed in partial fulfillment of the requirements of the D.Sc. degree from the Department of Health Policy and Management, Harvard School of Public Health, Boston.

6. Kidney Transplantation

1. National Center for Health Care Technology. 1981. *End-State Renal Disease: Pathophysiology, Dialysis, and Transplantation.* Rockville, MD: Office of Health Research, Statistics, and Technology, Public Health Service, U.S. Department of Health and Human Services.
2. Helper, T. 1989. *The Misfortunes of Others: End-State Renal Disease in the United Kingdom.* Cambridge, U.K.: Cambridge University Press.
3. Rettig, R. A., and Levinsky, N. G. (eds.). 1991. *Kidney Failure and the Federal Government.* Committee for the Study of the Medicare ESRD Program, Division of Health Care Services, Institute of Medicine. Washington, D.C.: National Academy Press.
4. Tilney, N. L. 1989. Renal transplantation. *Current Problems in Surgery* 26:601–669.
5. Kasiske, B. L., et al. 1991. The effect of race on access and outcome in transplantation. *New England Journal of Medicine* 324:302–307.
6. Dawidson, I. J. A., et al. 1990. Impact of race on renal transplant outcome. *Transplantation* 49:63–67.
7. Callender, C. O. 1989. The results of transplantation in blacks: Just the tip of the iceberg. *Transplantation Proceedings* 21:3407–3410.
8. Surmon, O. S. 1989. Psychiatric aspects of organ transplantation. *American Journal of Psychiatry* 146:972–982.

7. Epoetin Therapy for Renal Anemia

1. Rettig, R. A., and Levinsky, N. G. (eds.). 1991. *Kidney Failure and the Federal Government.* Committee for the Study of the Medicare ESRD Program, Divi-

sion of Health Care Services, Institute of Medicine. Washington, D.C.: National Academy Press.

2. Flaharty, K. K., Grimm, A. M., and Vlasses, P. H. 1989. Epoetin: Human recombinant erythropoietin. *Clinical Pharmacology* 8:769–782.

3. Eschbach, J. W., et al. 1989. USA multicenter clinical trial with recombinant human erythropoietin (Amgen): Results in hemodialysis patients. *Contributions to Nephrology* 76:160–165.

4. Eschbach, J. W., and Adamson, J. W. 1988. Correction of the anemia of hemodialysis (HD) in patients with recombinant human erythropoietin (r-HuEPO): Results of a multicenter study. *Kidney International* 33:189 (abstract).

5. Eschbach, J. W. 1990. Erythropoietin-associated hypertension. *New England Journal of Medicine* 323:999–1000.

6. Eschbach, J. W., et al. 1991. The safety of epoetin-alpha: Results of clinical trials in the United States. *Contributions to Nephrology* 88:72–80.

7. Epogen Package Insert. 1991. Amgen Inc.

8. Canadian Erythropoietin Study Group. 1990. Association between recombinant human erythropoietin and quality of life and exercise capacity of patients receiving haemodialysis. *British Medical Journal* 300:573–578.

9. Bergner, M., et al. 1981. The sickness impact profile: Development and final revision of a health status measure. *Medical Care* 18:787–805.

10. Patrick, D. L., and Deyo, R. A. 1989. Generic and disease-specific measures in assessing health status and quality of life. *Medical Care* 27(3 Suppl.):S217–S232.

11. Evans, R. W., Rader, B., Manninen, D. L., and the Cooperative Multicenter EPO Clinical Trial Group. 1990. The quality of life of hemodialysis recipients treated with recombinant human erythropoietin. *Journal of the American Medical Association* 263:825–830.

12. Lundin, A. P. 1989. Quality of life: Subjective and objective improvements with recombinant human erythropoietin. *Seminars in Nephrology* 9(1 Suppl. 1):22–29.

13. Tsai J.-C., et al. 1991. Clinical efficacy of recombinant human erythropoietin in the treatment of anemia in hemodialysis patients: Influence of dosing regimen, iron status and serum aluminum. *Kaoshiung Journal of Medical Science* 7:126–135.

14. Taylor, J., Henderson, I. S, and Mactier, R. A. 1991. Erythropoietin withdrawal. *British Medical Journal* 302:272–273.

15. Grimm, G., et al. 1990. Improvement of brain function in hemodialysis patients treated with erythropoietin. *Kidney International* 38:480–486.

16. Deniston, O. L., et al. 1990. Effect of long-term epoetin beta therapy on the quality of life of hemodialysis patients. *ASAIO Transactions* 36:M157–M160.

17. Graf, H., and Mayer, G. 1989. Clinical effects of partial correction of anemia using recombinant human erythropoietin on working capacity in dialysis patients. In Jelkmann, W., and Gross, A. J. (eds.), *Erythropoietin*, 156–164. New York: Springer-Verlag.

18. Human Resources Division. 1992. *Medicare: Millions in End-Stage Renal Disease Expenditures Shifted to Employer Health Plans*. Washington, D.C.: U.S. General Accounting Office, GAO/HRD-93-31.

19. Powe, N. R., et al. 1992. Access to recombinant erythropoietin by Medicare-entitled dialysis patients in the first year after FDA approval. *Journal of the American Medical Association* 268:1434–1440.
20. Eggers, Paul, Ph.D., Chief, Program Evaluation Branch, Health Care Financing Administration. Personal communication, March 16, 1992.
21. Sisk, J. E., Gianfrancesco, F. D., and Coster, J. M. 1991. Recombinant erythropoietin and Medicare payment. *Journal of the American Medical Association* 266:247–252.
22. *Federal Register,* September 4, 1991. 56(171):43706–43710.
23. Borzo, G. 1991. Dialysis market shifts to PD. *Health Industry Today* 54(5):1, 14–15.
24. Social Security Administration. 1991. *Disability.* Department of Health and Human Services. Baltimore: Social Security Administration Publication No. 05-10029.
25. Nissenson, F. R., for the National Cooperative rHu Erythropoietin Study Group. 1991. National Cooperative rHu Erythropoietin Study in patients with chronic renal failure: A phase IV multicenter study. *American Journal of Kidney Diseases* 18(4 Suppl. 1):24–33.

8. The Control of Postoperative Pain

1. Royal College of Surgeons of England, the College of Anesthetists. 1990. *Report of the Working Party on Pain after Surgery.* London: Royal College of Surgeons.
2. Cepeda, M. S., and Carr, D. B. 1993. The neuroendocrine response to postoperative pain. In Ferrante, F. M., and VadeBoncouer, T. (eds.), *Postoperative Pain Management,* 79–106. New York: Churchill Livingstone.
3. American Pain Society. 1989. *Principles of Analgesic Use in the Treatment of Acute Pain and Chronic Cancer Pain: A Concise Guide to Medical Practice,* 2nd ed. Skokie, IL: American Pain Society.
4. Kehlet, H. 1988. Modification of responses to surgery by neural blockage: Clinical implications. In Cousins, M. J., and Bridenbaugh, P. O. (eds.), *Neural Blockage in Clinical Anesthesia and Management of Pain,* 2nd ed., 145–188. Philadelphia: J. B. Lippincott.
5. Carr, D. B., et al. 1992. *Acute Pain Management: Operative or Medical Procedures and Trauma. Clinical Practice Guideline.* Rockville, MD: Agency for Health Care Policy and Research, Public Health Service, U.S. Department of Health and Human Services, AHCPR Pub. No. 92-0032.
6. Harmer, M., Rosen, M., and Vickers, M. D. 1985. *Patient-Controlled Analgesia.* Oxford: Blackwell Scientific Publications.
7. Cousins, M. J., and Phillips, G. D., (eds.). 1986. *Acute Pain Management.* New York: Churchill Livingstone Inc.
8. Wall, P. D. 1988. The prevention of postoperative pain. *Pain* 33:289–290.
9. Ballantyne, J. C., et al. 1993. Postoperative patient-controlled analgesia: Meta-analyses of initial randomized control trials. *Journal of Clinical Anesthesia* 5:182–193.

10. Ready, L. B., et al. 1988. Development of an anesthesiology-based postoperative pain service. *Anesthesiology* 68:100–106.
11. Bennett, R. L. 1985. Patient-controlled analgesia for the control of postoperative pain: Experience at the University of Kentucky. In Harmer, M., Rosen, M., and Vickers, M. D. (eds.), *Patient-Controlled Analgesia*, 149–155. Oxford: Blackwell Scientific Publications.
12. Melzack, R., and Wall, P. D. 1965. Pain mechanisms: A new theory. *Science* 10:971–979.
13. Devine, E. C., et al. 1988. Clinical and financial effects of psychoeducational care provided by staff nurses to adult surgical patients in the post-DRG environment. *American Journal of Public Health* 78:1293–1297.
14. Egbert, L. D., et al. 1964. Reduction of postoperative pain by encouragement and instruction of patients. *New England Journal of Medicine* 270:825–827.
15. Acute Pain Management Guideline Panel. In press. *Acute Pain Management: Operative or Medical Procedures and Trauma*, Technical Appendix. Rockville, MD: Agency for Health Care Policy and Research, Public Health Service, U.S. Department of Health and Human Services.
16. McCaffery, M., and Beebe, A. *Pain: Clinical Manual for Nursing Practice*. St. Louis: CV Mosby.
17. Jackson, D. 1989. A study of pain management: Patient controlled analgesia versus intramuscular analgesia. *Journal of Intravenous Nursing* 12:42–51.
18. Ready, L. B. 1991. Acute and postoperative pain services. *Pain Digest* 1:17–21.

9. Immunization against Measles

1. Katz, S. L., and Enders, J. F. 1965. Measles virus. In Horsfall, F. L., and Tamm, I. (eds.), *Viral and Rickettsial Infections of Man*, 4th ed., 784–801. Philadelphia: J. B. Lippincott.
2. Preblud, S. R., and Katz, S. L. 1988. Measles. In Plotkin, S. A., and Mortimer, E. A. (eds.), *Vaccines*, 182–222. Philadelphia: W. B. Saunders.
3. Bloch, A. B., et al. 1985. Health impact of measles vaccination in the United States. *Pediatrics* 76:524–532.
4. Hussey, G. D., and Klein, M. 1990. A randomized controlled trial of vitamin A in children with severe measles. *New England Journal of Medicine* 323:160–164.
5. Frieden, T. R., et al. 1992. Vitamin A levels and severity of measles: New York City. *American Journal of Diseases of Children* 146:182–186.
6. Hinman, A. R. 1988. Public health considerations. In Plotkin, S. A., and Mortimer, E. A. (eds.), *Vaccines*, 587–603. Philadelphia: W. B. Saunders.
7. Gindler, J. S., et al. 1992. The epidemiology of measles in the United States in 1989 and 1990. *Pediatric Infectious Disease Journal* 11:841–846.
8. Hersh, B. S., et al. 1992. The geographic distribution of measles in the United States, 1980 through 1989. *Journal of the American Medical Association* 267:1936–1941.
9. McConnochie, K. M., and Roghmann, K. J. 1992. Immunization opportunities missed among urban poor children. *Pediatrics* 89:1019–1026.

10. Hinman, A. R. 1990. Immunization in the United States. In *Child Health in 1990: The United States Compared to Canada, England and Wales, France, the Netherlands, and Norway. Supplement to Pediatrics* 86(Part 2):1064–1066.
11. King, G. E., et al. 1991. Clinical efficacy of measles vaccine during the 1990 measles epidemic. *Pediatric Infectious Disease Journal* 10:883–887.
12. Atkinson, W. L., Orenstein, W. A., and Krugman, S. 1992. The resurgence of measles in the United States, 1989–1990. *Annual Review of Medicine* 43:451–463.
13. The National Vaccine Advisory Committee. 1991. The measles epidemic: The problems, barriers, and recommendations. *Journal of the American Medical Association* 266:1547–1552.
14. Cutts, F. T., Orenstein, W. A., and Bernier, R. H. 1992. Causes of low pre-school immunization coverage in the United States. *Annual Review of Public Health* 385–398.

10. Treatment of Hypertension

1. Kannel, W. B., Schwartz, M. J., and McNamara, P. M. 1969. Blood pressure and risk of coronary heart disease: The Framingham study. *Diseases of the Chest* 56:43–52.
2. Kannel, W. B., et al. 1970. Epidemiologic assessment of the role of blood pressure in stroke: Framingham study. *Journal of the American Medical Association* 214:301–310.
3. Epstein, F. H., Ostrander, L. D., Jr., and Johnson, B. C. 1965. Epidemiological studies of cardiovascular disease in a total community—Tecumseh, Michigan. *Annals of Internal Medicine* 72:1170–1187.
4. Feinleib, M. 1984. Changes in cardiovascular epidemiology since 1950. *Bulletin of the New York Academy of Medicine* 60:449–464.
5. Drizd, T., Dannenberg, A. L., and Engel, A. 1986. *Vital and Health Statistics: Blood Pressure Levels in Persons 18–74 Years of Age in 1976–80, and Trends in Blood Pressure from 1960 to 1980 in the United States.* Hyattsville, MD: U.S. Department of Health and Human Services, Series 11, No. 234:36–39.
6. Feinleib, M. 1984. The magnitude and nature of decrease in coronary heart disease mortality rate. *American Journal of Cardiology* 54:2C–6C.
7. Freis, E. D., and the Veterans Administration Cooperative Study Group on Antihypertensive Agents. 1967. Effects of treatment on morbidity in hypertension. I. Results in patients with diastolic blood pressure average 115 through 129 mm Hg. *Journal of the American Medical Association* 202:1028–1034.
8. Freis, E. D., and the Veterans Administration Cooperative Study Group on Antihypertensive Agents. 1970. Effects of treatment on morbidity in hypertension. II. Results in patients with diastolic blood pressure average 90 through 114 mm Hg. *Journal of the American Medical Association* 213:1143–1152.
9. Freis, E. D., and the Veterans Administration Cooperative Study Group on Antihypertensive Agents. 1972. Effects of treatment on morbidity in hypertension. III. *Circulation* 45:991–1004.
10. Report of the Joint National Committee (JNC1) on the Detection, Evaluation,

and Treatment of High Blood Pressure: A cooperative study. 1977. *Journal of the American Medical Association* 237:255–261.

11. Hypertension Detection and Follow-up Program Cooperative Group. 1979. Five-year findings on the Hypertension Detection and Follow-up Program. 1. Reduction in mortality of persons with high blood pressure, including mild hypertension. *Journal of the American Medical Association* 242:2562–2571.

12. Hypertension Detection and Follow-up Program Cooperative Group. 1979. Five-year findings of Hypertension Detection and Follow-up Program. 2. Mortality by race, sex and age. *Journal of the American Medical Association* 242:2572–2577.

13. Feinleib, M., and Wilson, R. W. 1985. Trends in health in the United States. *Environmental Health Perspectives* 62:267–276.

14. MacMahon, S., et al. 1990. Epidemiology: Blood pressure, stroke, and coronary heart disease. Part 1, Prolonged differences in blood pressure: Prospective observational studies corrected for regression dilution bias. *Lancet* 335:765–774.

15. Stason, W. B. 1989. Cost and quality trade-offs in treatment of hypertension. *Hypertension* 13(5 Suppl.):I145–I148.

16. Veterans Administration Health Service Research and Development Service. 1984. *Effectiveness and Cost-effectiveness of the VA Pilot Hypertension Screening and Treatment Program. Final Report.* Washington, D.C.: Health Service Research and Development Service.

17. Weinstein, M. C., and Stason, W. B. 1976. *Hypertension: A Policy Perspective.* Cambridge, MA: Harvard University Press.

18. Littenberg, B., Garber, A. M., and Sox, H. C., Jr. 1990. Screening for hypertension. *Annals of Internal Medicine* 112:192–202.

19. The Gallup Organization Inc. 1986. *Gallup Survey of Hypertension Patients,* 1–41. Princeton: The Gallup Organization Inc.

20. Shulman, W. B., and Martinez, B. D. 1986. Financial cost as an obstacle to hypertension therapy. *American Journal of Public Health* 76:1105–1108.

21. Collins, R., et al. 1990. Epidemiology: Blood pressure, stroke and coronary heart disease. Part 2, Short-term reductions in blood pressure: Overview of randomised drug trials in their epidemiological context. *Lancet* 335:827–838.

22. Curtin, L. R., and Armstrong, R. J. 1988. *Decennial Life Tables for 1979–81. Volume 1, Number 2: United States Life Tables Eliminating Certain Causes of Death.* Center for Disease Control, Public Health Service, U.S. Department of Health and Human Services, DHHS Publication 1988, No. (PHS) 88:1150–1152.

11. The Contributions of Lenses to Visual Health

1. National Health Survey. 1978. *Refraction Status and Motility Defects of Persons 4–74 Years, United States, 1971–1972.* Hyattsville, MD: U.S. Department of Health, Education, and Welfare, HEW Publication No. (PHS) 78-1654.

2. Gregg, J. R. 1965. *The Story of Optometry.* New York: Ronald Press.

3. Bausch & Lomb Optical Co. 1950. *The Origin and History of Ophthalmic Lenses.*

4. Wertenbaker, L. T., and the Editors of U.S. News Books. 1981. *The Eye: Window to the World.* Washington, D.C.: U.S. News Books.

5. Curtin, B. J. 1985. *The Myopias.* New York: Harper and Row Publishers.

6. Curtin, B. J. 1970. Myopia: A review of its etiology, pathology, genesis, and treatment. *Survey of Ophthalmology* 15:1–17.

7. Pitts, D. 1982. Visual acuity as a function of age. *Journal of the American Optometric Association* 53:117–124.

8. Gittings, N. S., and Fozard, J. L. 1986. Age related changes in visual acuity. *Experimental Gerontology* 21:423–433.

9. Werner, D. L. 1981. The routine eye examination for the asymptomatic patient age 25–35. *Journal of the American Optometric Association* 52:899–903.

10. Sperduto, R. D., et al. 1983. Prevalence of myopia in the United States. *Archives of Ophthalmology* 101:405–407.

11. Yamane, S. J. 1990. Are hard lenses superior to soft? The advantages of soft lenses. *Cornea* 9(Suppl. 1):S12–S14; discussion, S15.

12. Public Health Service. 1990. *Healthy People 2000: National Health Promotion and Disease Prevention Objectives.* Washington, D.C.: Public Health Service, U.S. Department of Health and Human Services.

13. Thackray, J. 1984. High cost paid by industry for preventable eye injuries. *Occupational Health and Safety* 53:31–33.

14. Sheedy, J. E., et al. 1983. Recommended vision standards for police officers. *Journal of the American Optometric Association* 54:925–928.

15. McGee, F. 1979. New York City Police Academy. Cited in Sheedy, J. E., et al. 1983. Recommended vision standards for police officers. *Journal of the American Optometric Association* 54(10):925–928.

16. Good, G. W., and Augsburger, A. R. 1987. Uncorrected visual acuity standard for police applicants. *Journal of Police Science & Administration* 15:18–23.

17. California Department of Motor Vehicles. 1988. *Percent of California Driving Licenses with Vision Restrictions.* Personal communication.

18. Verbrugge, L. 1991. Physical and social disability in adults. *Primary care research: Theory and methods: Conference Proceedings,* 31–35. Rockville, MD: Agency for Health Care Policy and Research, Public Health Service, U.S. Department of Health and Human Services.

19. Gordon, A., and Crooks, C. T. 1988. Optometric services and private health insurance. *Journal of the American Optometric Association* 59:62–70.

20. Butler, J. A., et al. 1985. Medical care use and expenditure among children and youth in the United States: Analysis of a national probability sample. *Pediatrics* 76:495–507.

21. Lurie, N., et al. 1989. How free care improved vision in the health insurance experiment. *American Journal of Public Health* 79:640–642.

22. Milne, J. S. 1970. Longitudinal studies of vision in older people. *Age and Ageing* 8:160–166.

23. Stone, D. H., and Shannon, D. J. 1978. Screening for impaired visual acuity in middle age in general practice. *British Medical Journal* 2:859–861.

24. Stults, B. M. 1984. Preventive health care for the elderly. *Western Journal of Medicine* 141:832–845.

12. Dentistry

1. National Institute of Dental Research. 1989. *Oral Health of United States Children, The National Survey of Dental Caries in U.S. School Children: 1986–1987, National and Regional Findings.* NIH Publication No. 89–2247. Bethesda: National Institutes of Health.
2. Burt, B. A., and Eklund, S. A. 1992. *Dentistry, Dental Practice, and the Community,* 4th ed. Philadelphia: W. B. Saunders.
3. Pendrys, D. G., and Stamm, J. W. 1990. Relationship of total fluoride intake to beneficial effects and enamel fluorosis. *Journal of Dental Research* 69 (Special Issue):529–538.
4. Ad Hoc Subcommittee on Fluoride. 1991. *Review of Fluoride Benefits and Risks. Report of the Ad Hoc Subcommittee on Fluoride of the Committee to Coordinate Environmental Health and Related Programs.* Washington, D.C.: Public Health Service, Department of Health and Human Services.
5. National Institute of Dental Research. 1987. *Oral Health of United States Adults, The National Survey of Oral Health in U.S. Employed Adults and Seniors: 1985–1986. National Findings.* NIH Publication No. 87–2868. Bethesda: National Institutes of Health.
6. Burt, B. A. 1978. Influences for change in the dental health status of populations: An historical perspective. *Journal of Public Health Dentistry* 38:262–288.
7. Reisine, S. T. 1985. Dental health and public policy: The social impact of dental disease. *American Journal of Public Health* 75:27–30.
8. Levit, K. R., et al. 1992. National health expenditures, 1990. *Health Care Financing Review* 13:29–52.
9. Bowen, W. H. 1991. Dental caries: Is it an extinct disease? *Journal of the American Dental Association* 122:49–52.
10. Mertz-Fairhurst, E. J. 1992. Pit-and-fissure sealants: A global lack of science transfer? *Journal of Dental Research* 71:1543–1544.

13. Total Joint Replacement for the Treatment of Osteoarthritis

1. Liang, M. H., and Fortin, P. 1991. Management of osteoarthritis of the hip and knee. *New England Journal of Medicine* 325:125–127.
2. Wilson, M. G., et al. 1990. Idiopathic symptomatic osteoarthritis of the hip and knee: A population-based incidence study. *Mayo Clinic Proceedings* 65:1214–1221.
3. Selman, S. W. 1989. Impact of total hip replacement on quality of life. *Orthopaedic Nursing* 8:43–49.
4. Arthritis Foundation. 1983. *Arthritis: Surgery Information to Consider.* Atlanta: Arthritis Foundation.

5. Quam, J. P., et al. 1991. Total knee arthroplasty: A population-based study. *Mayo Clinic Proceedings* 66:589–595.

6. McInnes, J., et al. 1992. A controlled evaluation of continuous passive motion in patients undergoing total knee arthroplasty. *Journal of the American Medical Association* 268:1423–1428.

7. Hoffinger, S. A., Keggi, K. J., and Zatorske, L. E. 1991. Primary ceramic hip replacement: A prospective study of 119 hips. *Orthopedics* 14:523–531.

8. Windsor, R. E. 1991. Management of total knee arthroplasty infection. *Orthopedic Clinics of North America* 22:531–538.

9. Echeverri, A., Shelley, P., and Wroblewski, B. M. 1988. Long term results of hip arthroplasty for failure of previous surgery. *Journal of Bone and Joint Surgery* 70B:49–51.

10. Kaempffe, F. A., Lifeso, R. M., and Meinking, C. 1991. Intermittent pneumatic compression versus coumadin: Prevention of deep vein thrombosis in lower-extremity total joint arthroplasty. *Clinical Orthopaedics and Related Research* 269:89–97.

11. Stulberg, B. N., et al. 1984. Deep vein thrombosis following total knee replacement. *Journal of Bone and Joint Surgery* 66A:194–201.

12. Newington, D. P., Bannister, G. C., and Fordyce, M. 1990. Primary total hip replacement in patients over 80 years of age. *Journal of Bone and Joint Surgery* 72B:450–452.

13. Rand, A., and Ilstrup, D. M. 1991. Survivorship analysis of total knee arthroplasty: Cumulative rates of survival of 9200 total knee arthroplasties. *Journal of Bone and Joint Surgery* 73A:397–409.

14. Krugluger, J., et al. 1991. Longterm analysis of Sheehan total knee arthroplasty. *International Orthopaedics* 15:149–154.

14. Peptic Ulcer

1. Hirschowitz, B. I., et al. 1958. Demonstration of a new gastroscope, the "fiberscope." *Gastroenterology* 35:50–53.

2. Chalmers, T. C., Reitman, D., and Schroeder, B. 1980. Emergency diagnosis and treatment of gastrointestinal hemorrhage. In Barany, F. R., Shields, R., and Caprilli, O. (eds.), *Gastrointestinal Emergencies 2: Proceedings of the Second International Symposium on Gastrointestinal Emergencies: Rome (June 7–8 1979)*. Oxford: Pergamon.

3. Sippy, B. W. 1915. Gastric and duodenal ulcer. *Journal of the American Medical Association* 64:1625–1630.

4. Chalmers, T. C. 1974. The impact of controlled trials on the practice of medicine. *Mount Sinai Journal of Medicine* 41:753–759.

5. Chalmers, T. C., et al. 1988. Data analysis in gastroenterology: Vagotomy for recurrent duodenal ulcer. *Gastroenterology International* 1:41–48.

6. Hentschel, E., et al. 1993. Effect of ranitidine and amoxicillin plus metronidazole on the eradication of *Helicobacter pylori* and the recurrence of duodenal ulcer. *New England Journal of Medicine* 328:308–312.

15. Oral Contraceptives

1. Baird, D. T., and Glasier, A. F. 1993. Hormonal contraception. *New England Journal of Medicine* 328:1543–1549.
2. Tietze, C. 1977. New estimates of mortality associated with fertility control. *Family Planning Perspectives* 9:74–76.
3. Rawson, N. S. B., Pearce, G. L., and Inman, W. H. W. 1990. Prescription-event monitoring: Methodology and recent progress. *Journal of Clinical Epidemiology* 43:509–522.

16. Surgery and Anesthesiology

1. Welch, C. E. 1992. *A Twentieth Century Surgeon: My Life in the Massachusetts General Hospital,* 295–296. Boston: Massachusetts General Hospital, distributed by Watson Publishing International (ISBN 0-88135-182-2).
2. Bunker, J. P., Barnes, B. A., and Mosteller, F. (eds.). 1977. *Costs, Risks, and Benefits of Surgery,* xiii–xvii, 223–239, 246–261, 372–384. New York: Oxford University Press.
3. Milamed, D. R., and Hedley-Whyte, J. 1994. Contributions of the surgical sciences to reduction of mortality in the United States, 1968–1988. *Annals of Surgery* 219:94–102.
4. Treves, F. 1900. Address in surgery: The surgeon in the nineteenth century. *British Medical Journal* 2:285–289.
5. Lancaster, H. O. 1990. The role of therapy in the decline of mortality. In Lancaster, H. O. (ed.), *Expectations of Life,* 453–476. New York: Springer-Verlag.
6. American College of Surgeons and the American Surgical Association. 1975. *Surgery in the United States: A Summary Report of the Study on Surgical Services for the United States,* 11–15, 155–157. Chicago: American College of Surgeons and American Surgical Association.
7. Rutkow, I. 1986. Urological operations in the United States: 1979 to 1984. *Journal of Urology* 135:1206–1208.
8. Eichhorn, J. H., et al. 1986. Standards for patient monitoring during anesthesia at Harvard Medical School. *Journal of the American Medical Association* 256:1017–1020.
9. Eichhorn, J. H. 1989. Prevention of intraoperative anesthesia accidents and related severe injury through safety monitoring. *Anesthesiology* 70:572–577.
10. American Society of Anesthesiologists. 1994. Basic standards for preanesthesia care, 734; Standards for basic anesthetic monitoring, 735–736; Standards for postanesthesia care, 737–738. In *1994 Directory of Members.* Park Ridge, IL: American Society of Anesthesiologists.
11. Berenson, R. A. 1984. Intensive care units (ICUs): Clinical outcomes, costs and decisionmaking (Health Technology Case Study 28). Washington, D.C.: Office of Technology Assessment, U. S. Congress, OTA-HCS-28.
12. Ermann, D. 1988. Surgery and the changing system of health care delivery. In

Frankel, M. L. (ed.), *Surgical Care in the United States: A Policy Perspective,* 125–143. Baltimore: Johns Hopkins University Press.

17. Improving the Health Care System

1. Chalmers, I., Enking, M., and Keirse, M. J. N. C. 1989. *Effective Care in Pregnancy and Childbirth.* Oxford: Oxford University Press.
2. Chalmers, I. 1988. *The Oxford Database of Perinatal Trials.* Oxford: Oxford University Press.
3. Enkin, M., Keirse, M. J. N. C., and Chalmers, I. 1989. *A Guide to Effective Care in Pregnancy and Childbirth.* Oxford: Oxford University Press.
4. Office of Medical Applications of Research. 1990. *Health Care Delivery Research Using Hospital Firms: Workshop Summary, April 30–May 1.* Bethesda: Office of Medical Applications of Research, National Institutes of Health, Public Health Service.
5. Neuhauser, D. 1991. Research on the delivery of medical care using hospital firms. *Medical Care* 29 (Supplement):JS1a–JS70.
6. Neuhauser, D. 1992. Progress in firms research. *International Journal of Technology Assessment in Health Care* 8:321–324.
7. Neuhauser, D. 1989. The Metro firm trials and ongoing patient randomization. In J. M. Tanur et al. (eds.), *Statistics: A Guide to the Unknown,* 3rd ed., 25–30. Pacific Grove: Wadsworth and Brooks/Cole Advanced Books and Software.
8. Adams, M. E., et al. 1992. Economic analysis in randomized control trials. *Medical Care* 30:231–243.
9. Patrick, D. L., and Erickson, P. 1993. *Health Status and Health Policy: Quality of Life in Health Care Evaluation and Resource Allocation.* New York: Oxford University Press.
10. Gilbert, J. P., McPeek, B., and Mosteller, F. 1977. Statistics and ethics in surgery and anesthesia. *Science* 198:684–689.

18. Innovation-Specific Improvements

1. Office of Technology Assessment. 1992. *Evaluation of the Oregon Medicaid Proposal.* Office of Technology Assessment, U.S. Congress. Washington, D.C.: U.S. Government Printing Office, OTA-H531.

Acknowledgments

Chapter 4

Permission is granted from the authors and the managing editor of *Ophthalmology* to quote from J. C. Javitt et al., "Detecting and treating retinopathy in patients with type I diabetes mellitus: A health policy model," *Ophthalmology* 97 (1990):483–495.

Chapter 5

Quotations from *Darkness Visible* by William Styron: Copyright © 1990 by William Styron. Reprinted by permission of Random House, Inc.

Table 5-1: Adapted from *Diagnostic and Statistical Manual of Mental Disorders,* 3rd ed., Revised (Washington, D.C.: American Psychiatric Association, 1987), with permission from the American Psychiatric Association.

Figure 5-1: Data from D. Neville and M. C. Weinstein, "Lifetime costs and health consequences of an incident case of major depressive disorder," unpublished manuscript, 1989, cited with permission from the authors.

Table 5-3: Cited from D. Neville, "Program evaluation: An illustration of three quantitative approaches in the field of health promotion," D.Sc. dissertation, Harvard School of Public Health, 1989, with permission from the author.

Chapter 6

It is a pleasure to acknowledge the help of Theodore I. Steinman in developing the patient vignettes.

Chapter 7

Paul W. Eggers granted permission to use data on Medicare utilization and expenditures for erythropoietin in the end stage renal disease population.

The author wishes to express appreciation for advice and information from Paul W. Eggers and Walter Eichner in the preparation of this chapter.

Chapter 8

Figure 8-1: Data adapted from Table 1 of the *Report of the Working Party on Pain after Surgery* (1990) by permission of The Royal College of Surgeons of England.

Figure 8-2: Reproduced from Figure 2.12 in M. J. Cousins and G. D. Phillips, *Acute Pain Management* (New York: Churchill Livingston Inc., 1986), with permission from Churchill Livingstone Inc.

Figure 8-3: Reproduced from Figure 10.6 in R. L. Bennett, "Patient-controlled analgesia for the control of postoperative pain: Experience at the University of Kentucky," in M. Harmer, M. Rosen, and M. D. Vickers (eds.), *Patient-Controlled Analgesia* (Oxford: Blackwell Scientific Publications, 1985), with permission from Blackwell Scientific Publications Limited.

Chapter 9

The Cambridge University Press gave permission to reproduce the copyrighted material on the Children's Vaccine Initiative on page 134.

Chapter 11

The authors wish to thank the following people for their assistance with the preparation of this manuscript: Daniel M. Albert, Michael Breton, Larry Clausen, Judith Singer, David Guyton, Lee Regan, Firmon Hardenbergh, Mary Janke, Carl Pierchala, L. Shulman, Thomas Chalmers, John Hedley-Whyte, and the staff of the California Department of Motor Vehicles.

Tables 11-1 and 11-2: Data from N. S. Gittings and J. L. Fozard, "Age related changes in visual acuity," *Experimental Gerontology* 21(1986):423–433, used with permission from Pergamon Press Ltd, Headington Hill Hall, Oxford OX3 OBW.

Table 11-4: Permission from the *Annual Review of Public Health* to reproduce material from L. M. Verbrugge, "Recent, present, and future health of American adults," in L. Breslow and J. E. Fielding (eds.), *Annual Review of Public Health* 10(1989):333–361.

Chapter 12

The authors would like to thank Brian Burt, Jane Weintraub, and Alex White for their helpful comments on this manuscript.

Chapter 15

Table 15-1: Based on data used with the permission of The Alan Guttmacher Institute from Christopher Tietze, "New estimates of mortality associated with fertility control," *Family Planning Perspectives,* vol. 9, no. 2, March/April 1977.

Chapter 16

Quotation on page 223 from Claude E. Welch, M.D., S.D., *A Twentieth Century Surgeon: My Life in the Massachusetts General Hospital* (Boston: Massachusetts General Hospital, distributed by Watson Publishing International [ISBN 0-88135-182-2], 1992), pp. 295–296, used with permission from the author, the Massachusetts General Hospital, and Watson Publishing International.

Figures 16-1, 16-3–7: Adapted from D. R. Milamed and J. Hedley-Whyte, "Contributions of the surgical sciences to reduction of mortality in the United States, 1968–1988," *Annals of Surgery* 219(1994):94–102, with permission from the publisher.

Chapter 17

Some of the materials in this chapter were originally presented in a somewhat different form in F. Mosteller, "Some evaluation needs," in K. S. Warren and F. Mosteller (eds.), *Doing More Good Than Harm: The Evaluation of Health Care Interventions* (Annals of the New York Academy of Sciences, vol. 703; New York: New York Academy of Sciences, 1993). 12–17. The New York Academy of Sciences gave permission for this use.

Chapter 18

Some of the material in this chapter was originally described in a somewhat different form in F. Mosteller and H. Frazier, "Improving the contributions of technology assessment to the health care system of the U.S.A.," *Journal of the Italian Statistical Society* 1(1992):297–310. The adaptation for presentation in this volume appears with the permission of the editor of the *Journal of the Italian Statistical Society.*

About the Authors

Miriam E. Adams, Sc.D., 36 Garfield Street, Cambridge, Massachusetts, 02138, previously a Research Associate in Health Policy and Management at the Harvard School of Public Health, is now studying Clinical Social Work at the Simmons College School of Social Work. Her research interests include the effectiveness, safety, and economic costs of medical and mental health technologies, and patients' understanding of the potential risks and benefits of their treatments.

Daniel M. Albert, M.D., is the Frederick A. Davis Professor of Ophthalmology and Chairman, Department of Ophthalmology, University of Wisconsin, School of Medicine, 600 Highland Avenue, Madison, Wisconsin, 53792. His interests include clinical ophthalmology and clinical and experimental eye pathology, and his research focuses on studies of the cause and treatment of eye disease using transgenic mouse models.

Michael R. Albert, B.A., University of Massachusetts Medical School, Box 504, 55 Lake Avenue North, Worcester, Massachusetts, 01655, is currently a medical student with research interest in experimental studies on the retina.

Alexia Antczak-Bouckoms, D.M.D., Sc.D., M.P.H., is Lecturer in Dental Public Health, Harvard School of Public Health, 677 Huntington Avenue, Boston, Massachusetts, 02115. In her research, Antczak-Bouckoms applies a variety of analytic methods for assessment of technologies and development of health policy to a wide range of oral health conditions.

Jane C. Ballantyne, M.D., is Clinical and Research Fellow in Anesthetics and Pain, Department of Anesthesia, Massachusetts General Hospital, Fruit Street, Boston, Massachusetts, 02114. Her primary clinical interest is the treatment of acute, chronic, and cancer pain. In her research on the evaluation of pain treatments, she utilizes data from multiple trials and, in particular, meta-analysis of available data.

Elisabeth Burdick, M.S., is Research Statistician in the Department of Health Policy and Management, Harvard School of Public Health, 677 Huntington Avenue, Boston, Massachusetts, 02115. Her work focuses on medical technology assessment, meta-analysis, and uses of medical registry data.

Daniel B. Carr, M.D., is Saltonstall Professor of Pain Research, Department of Anesthesiology and Medicine, Tufts University School of Medicine, and Anesthetist, New England Medical Center, 750 Washington Street, Boston, Massachusetts, 02111. Formerly the Director of the Massachusetts General Hospital Pain Center, Carr has research interests in opioid analgesics, and he co-chaired the federal panels that prepared clinical practice guidelines for acute pain management and cancer pain management.

Thomas C. Chalmers, M.D., of 32 Pinewood Village, West Lebanon, New Hampshire, 03784, is Adjunct Professor of Medicine, Tufts University School of Medicine; Adjunct Lecturer, Department of Health Policy and Management, Harvard School of Public Health; and Adjunct Lecturer, Department of Epidemiology and Biostatistics, Boston University School of Medicine. He devotes his time to the planning, conduct, and reporting of meta-analyses of clinical trials, diagnostic evaluations, and epidemiologic studies.

Graham A. Colditz, M.B.B.S., Dr.P.H., is Associate Professor of Medicine, Harvard Medical School, and Associate Professor of Epidemiology at Harvard School of Public Health. His research interests include the relations between hormones and cancer among women and those between life-style and health. He also studies and applies methods of meta-analysis to issues in public health.

Howard S. Frazier, M.D., is Professor of Medicine, Harvard Medical School, and Professor in the Department of Health Policy and Management, Harvard School of Public Health, 677 Huntington Avenue, Boston, Massachusetts, 02115. His research interests include the assessment of medical technology and the development of methods for evaluating the quality of ambulatory care.

Leon D. Goldman, M.D., is Assistant Professor in Surgery, Harvard Medical School, and Surgeon, Beth Israel Hospital, 330 Brookline Avenue, Boston, Massachusetts, 02215. He is the Director of Laparoscopic and Endoscopic Surgery for the Department of Surgery at the Beth Israel Hospital.

John Hedley-Whyte, M.D., is the David S. Sheridan Professor of Anaesthesia and Respiratory Therapy, Harvard University; Professor in the Department of Health Policy and Management, Harvard School of Public Health; and Professor in the Department of Veterans Affairs Medical Center, Brockton/West Roxbury, 1400 VFW Parkway, Boston, Massachusetts, 02132. He has contributed to the assessment of surgical outcomes and medical technology, and to the development of national and international voluntary consensus standards for medical devices and care.

Ada Jacox, R.N., Ph.D., is Independence Foundation Chair in Health Policy, The Johns Hopkins University School of Nursing, 1830 East Monument Street, Baltimore, Maryland, 21205. Her research interests include the development of clinical practice guidelines for pain management and determining factors that influence nursing care costs and patient outcomes.

Sidney Klawansky, M.D., Ph.D., is Lecturer, Technology Assessment Group, Department of Health Policy and Management, Harvard School of Public Health, 677 Huntington Avenue, Boston, Massachusetts, 02115. In his studies of how a variety of medical conditions—such as breast cancer, hypertension, obesity, and drug dependence—respond over time to intervention, he is developing methods to improve our ability to use short-term data from therapeutic interventions to predict long-term outcomes.

Marie-A McPherson, M.B.A., Technology Assessment Group, Harvard School of Public Health, 677 Huntington Avenue, Boston, Massachusetts, 02115, is engaged in research on the regulatory and diffusion aspects of medical technologies.

Donna Mahrenholz, R.N., Ph.D., is Assistant Professor and Research Associate, Graduate Academic Programs, The Johns Hopkins School of Nursing, 1830 East Monument Street, Baltimore, Maryland, 21205. Her research focuses on methods to evaluate scientific evidence, the relationship of costs of care to patient outcomes and patient satisfaction, and the development of methods to assess clinical outcomes.

Georgianna Marks, M.S., R.N., C.S., is Clinical Nurse Specialist, Beth Israel Hospital, 330 Brookline Avenue, Boston, Massachusetts, 02215, with a research interest in quality-of-life issues. Her current work deals with end-of-life ethical decisionmaking, advance directives, and health care proxy education and information.

Donald N. Medearis, Jr., M.D., is the Charles Wilder Professor of Pediatrics, Harvard Medical School, and Chief, Children's Service, Massachusetts General Hospital, Ellison 1934, Fruit Street, Boston, Massachusetts, 02114, whose clinical and research interests are the infectious diseases of children; his particular concern is the unmet needs of children.

Debra R. Milamed, M.S., is Associate in Anaesthesia, Harvard Medical School and the Department of Veterans Affairs Medical Center, Brockton/West Roxbury, 1400 VFW Parkway, Boston, Massachusetts, 02132, has participated in research on the assessment of medical technology and the development of methods for the evaluation of surgical practice. As Secretary of several subcommittees of the American Society for Testing and Materials' Committee F-29 on Anesthetic and Respiratory Equipment, she is involved in the development of national voluntary consensus standards for these devices.

Frederick Mosteller, Ph.D., is Roger I. Lee Professor of Mathematical Statistics, Emeritus, Harvard School of Public Health, 677 Huntington Avenue, Boston, Massachusetts, 02115. He carries out assessments of medical technologies and studies methods of doing research synthesis, especially meta-analysis. His recent work, in the Department of Statistics, Harvard University, deals with exploratory data analysis and the analysis of variance.

Jennifer F. Taylor, Ph.D., is Clinical Fellow in Psychology in the Department of Psychiatry, Harvard Medical School, Cognitive Behavior Therapy Unit, McLean Hospital, 115 Mill Street, Belmont, Massachusetts, 02178. Her research interests include the assessment of medical technologies and quality of life, and behavioral medicine.

J. F. C. Tulloch, B.D.S., B.Orth., F.B.S., R.C.S., is an Assistant Professor of Orthodontics at the University of North Carolina Dental School at Chapel Hill, North Carolina. In her research on technology assessment and decision analysis, she has evaluated alternative extraction policies for third molar teeth and is currently conducting a randomized, controlled clinical trial of early intervention in orthodontics.

Janice Ulmer, R.N., Ph.D., is Assistant Professor, The Johns Hopkins School of Nursing, 1830 East Baltimore Street, Baltimore, Maryland, 21205. Her major activities are in the development of clinical guidelines for management of acute pain and cancer pain under the aegis of the Agency for Health Care Policy and Research.

Grace Wyshak, Ph.D., is Lecturer on Psychiatry, Harvard Medical School, and on Biostatistics and Population and International Health, Harvard School of Public Health, 665 Huntington Avenue, Boston, Massachusetts, 02115. Her research interests include application and development of biostatistical methods in women's health, twinning and multiple births, methodological and applied statistics in psychiatry, cross-cultural psychiatry and human rights, health promotion, and technology assessment.

Index